SLIM

forever

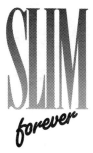

SLIM
forever

Robert Harris D.C.

SUNSHINE
PUBLICATIONS

SLIM FOREVER
Robert Harris
A Sunshine Publications Book

First published in Australia September 1993 by

Sunshine Publications
P.O. Box 3669
Parramatta NSW 2124
Australia

First reprint November 1993
Second reprint June 1994

National Library of Australia Cataloguing-in-Publication data:

Harris, Robert 1938

SLIM FOREVER

ISBN 0 646 14249 6

Research and design coordination by Jennifer Harris
Cover art by Fred Hawkesley
Cartoons by Caroline Magerl
Photography by Mike Thorpe
Typesetting by Graphic Partners

Printed in Hong Kong by Kings Time Printing Press Ltd.

NOTICE TO READERS

WARNING

THE AUTHOR

Robert Harris has been a health care professional for almost 20 years. He graduated from Palmer College of Chiropractic in the United States with the degree of Doctor of Chiropractic, and is currently undertaking doctoral studies in Human Development with The Fielding Institute, Santa Barbara, California.

'I spent much of my adult life fighting a weight problem. Failed attempts at dieting prompted me to seek answers to why we gain and retain unwanted body fat.

Slim Forever is the culmination of a seven year commitment to research, and the development of a weight loss and weight maintenance program that is effective, safe and sustainable. But the benefits of consuming a balanced diet extend beyond helping those who suffer from being overweight or obesity. The ability of this program to unlock stored body fat for the production of energy will ensure athletes, and those who are already slim, enjoy an increase in endurance and general well-being.

The program has enabled me to lose 25 kg [55 lb] of excess fat and replace most of it with solid muscle. I can now control my weight without depriving myself of good food or a social drink and at 55 I believe I am fitter, stronger and more energetic than I have been in 30 years.

I take great pleasure in sharing the *Slim Forever* program with you'.

contents

part III

THE WAY

introduction

If you would like to lose weight and keep it off without depriving yourself of good food and perhaps a social drink, this book will be your salvation.

The *Slim Forever* program is not a diet. It is a lifelong commitment to balanced eating, developed to allow you to rid yourself of unwanted body fat and keep it off *forever*. But, losing weight is not just about how you look. Losing weight is about feeling good about yourself, about being happier, about being more energetic, and last but certainly not least about living longer. Your *Slim Forever* experience will be your passport to a new level of physical and mental vitality enabling you to participate in life and enjoy it to the fullest.

If you are to achieve your goal of being slimmer some of your eating habits will have to change, but change in this case does not mean isolation from many of your favourite foods. By following this program you will find the changes in the quality and the quantity of the food you eat to be surprisingly pleasant and very satisfying.

Hunger does not form part of the *Slim Forever* process. By coincidence, the most fattening foods are invariably the foods which fail to satisfy your hunger and in many cases actually increase your level of perceived hunger. By decreasing your intake of hunger stimulating and fattening foods and increasing your intake of satisfying and body building foods you will control both your appetite and your overall weight.

This book will examine many of the current dietary myths and the sometimes incorrect postulations so frequently reinforced by a bombardment of advertising and misinformation generously sponsored by self-serving food manufacturers. You will be invited to consider new evidence in support of such controversial issues as:

- why fresh dietary fats are not the cause of elevated blood cholesterol;
- why red meat is an excellent food source; and
- why the eating of grains and cereals may be doing you more harm than good.

With you the reader in mind, this book has been presented in a different and easy to use format. All the information necessary to get you started on your **weight loss** program is presented in the front of the book where it belongs, instead of hidden behind hundreds of pages of preamble which is often more difficult to digest than the diet itself. You will of course want to know more about how your body functions and why *Slim Forever* is the safest, and perhaps the only scientifically sound, weight loss and weight maintenance program yet developed. This you may do by referring to the informative chapters contained in Part II. Each chapter deals with a specific topic of physiological and nutritional interest written in a manner you will understand. These topics are not presented in any specific order of priority and the reading of one chapter is not a prerequisite to the reading of another. Once you get started on your *Slim Forever* program you may at your convenience randomly access the topics you personally consider to be most important and in the order you wish to read them. In this easy to read format this book will scientifically address the causes, the effects and the remedies of the conditions of being overweight and obesity.

This text may appear to contradict some of your present attitudes and opinions regarding dietary health, but please keep an open mind until you have read this book in its entirety. The facts will speak for themselves. Your new understanding of how your body functions and how it reacts to the foods you eat may well add many active and pleasurable years to your life.

Welcome to *Slim Forever*.

part I

THE HOW

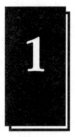

1

your personal weight loss program

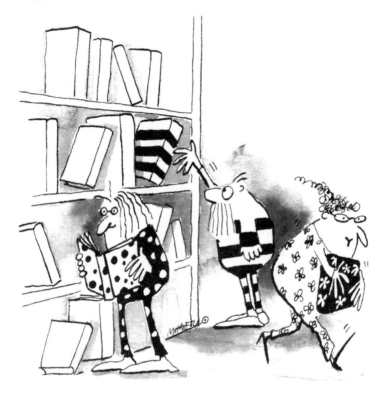

*Man's sustenance must be suited to the laws
that govern his body. Our ability to adapt
cannot stretch beyond narrow limits.*

S. Giedion

The *Slim Forever* program consists of two distinct parts. The first part, the **weight loss** program, will enable you to lose unwanted body fat without the threat of starvation and muscle wasting common to most commercial diets. This you will achieve by supplying your body with just the right balance of essential vitamins, minerals, proteins and fresh fats necessary for good health, but with a controlled reduction in carbohydrates. By balancing your food intake your body will switch from your current fat creation and storage mode to releasing stored fat for the production of energy, and you will safely and surely reduce your overall burden of unwanted body weight.

When you reach your desired level of fat loss, and you may stop at any time you want, you will move to the second part, the **weight maintenance** program. This will enable you to increase your carbohydrate intake and still maintain your new-found levels of good health and slimness.

Most commercial diets recommend meals such as 5 oz/140 g of skinned boiled chicken together with a salad of perhaps lettuce with tomato and a piece of fruit without any apparent consideration given to the relative size of the person undertaking the diet. There can be no argument that it takes more energy to move a large object than it does to move a small object of similar density. This being the case, simple logic dictates that the basic daily food and energy requirements of a naturally larger framed person will usually be greater than those of a naturally smaller framed person. Similarly, the need for body building protein is greater in a person with a naturally larger body simply because of an increase in the mass of functional tissue. As all body tissue is in a constant state of breaking down and rebuilding, the more tissue there is to replace, the greater will be the demand for body building protein. Consequently, any person undertaking an effective weight loss or weight maintenance program must consume quantities of the various food groups specifically tailored to satisfy his or her particular daily nutrient requirements.

To achieve your goal you will need to customise your personal daily intake allowance of protein and carbohydrate for both the **weight loss** and the **weight maintenance** portions of your program. This you may readily do by referring to the *Protein and carbohydrate assessment charts* appearing later in this chapter. Nothing could be easier.

Once you have established your optimum personal daily intake allowance of the two major food groups, protein and carbohydrate, an enormous array of exciting and satisfying meals will be at your disposal. Contrary to popular belief, losing weight does not mean you must eat microscopic meals of boring and tasteless food which traditionally leave you feeling hungry and light-headed. The foods you will eat with the *Slim Forever* program will not necessarily differ greatly from the foods you are eating right now, and you will not be required to spend your hard earned cash on expensive prepared foods or appetite suppressors. You will eat satisfying and tasty foods readily available from your local supermarket or from the menu of your favourite restaurant. The trick is not so much what you eat, but rather what quantities of the three major food groups, protein, carbohydrate and fat, you consume and when. If you can face the prospect of an evening meal such as steak, a baked potato with butter or sour cream, a salad and perhaps a glass of wine, you are as good as slim right now.

Just how much fat a person should or should not eat is a dilemma. As fat is often a hidden component of the food we eat, you will not be required to specifically calculate your daily fat intake by weight or volume. To ensure you are including just the right amount of fat and oils in your diet, a simple rule of thumb to measure fat intake will be outlined later in this chapter.

In determining your specific levels of allowable food intake it is important that you calculate your very own personal **weight loss** and **weight maintenance** programs using your body weight as it should be and not what it is at this point in time. This is achieved by establishing your **lean body weight**, a term best described as the sum of your fat-free body weight together with a reasonable and healthy level of body fat. Our individual lean body weights remain relatively constant throughout our adult lives, but the amount of surplus fat a body may carry can vary greatly from person to person, or even from year to year in the same person.

Muscle, blood, skin and bone require an ongoing supply of body building nutrients in order to sustain the life process. Not so your stored body fat. Body fat is a rather inert mass which just hangs around getting in the way, and, although it does not require feeding, it will continue to increase in volume if you persist in eating an overabundance of fat forming food.

Given it is only active body tissue that requires nutritional sustenance, the inclusion of your excess body fat in your lean body weight calculations would have you consuming quantities of food far in excess of your optimum daily requirements. For example, if your lean body weight is 140 lb/64 kg, but your current total body weight is 175 lb/80 kg, you would customise your program using the 140 lb/64 kg weight, not the 175 lb/80 kg weight. To do otherwise would have you eating 20% more food than your body requires and you would not only fail in your attempt to lose weight, you would probably continue to gain unwanted body fat.

DETERMINING YOUR LEAN BODY WEIGHT

Determining your lean body weight is a very simple exercise. Most of us achieve full physical maturity by the time we reach age 20 years, and this is the weight you will use as the basis for your personal program calculations. Do not be alarmed. It is not suggested you should necessarily return to the weight you were when you were 20 years old, although you could if you so desire, but this is an ideal starting point in establishing your optimum daily intake levels of the various food groups.

If you consider you were either overweight or underweight at age 20 years, simply add or subtract the amount of weight you think would have been appropriate to put you at your ideal weight at the time and use the amended figure as your lean body weight.

There is good reason for using your actual or amended body weight at age 20 years as a starting point. The *Slim Forever* program was tested with a number of control groups and it was discovered that, almost without exception, every person interviewed underestimated the extent of his or her excess of body fat by somewhere between one-half and two-thirds. For example, if you consider yourself to be 10 lb/4.5 kg overweight your real fatty excess is more likely to be somewhere between 20 lb/9 kg and 30 lb/13.5 kg. In arbitrarily assessing our own levels of fatty excess we have a tendency to concentrate only on the most obvious areas of fat deposition.

The primary sites of visible fat formation on the female are the buttocks and upper thighs, and on the male the abdominal and lower back areas. But, as body fat forms it spreads outwards and sideways, a process resulting in more widespread fat distribution than most of us imagine.

Many of us adopt the attitude that a little fat on the arms and legs is acceptable, but a loss of 10 lb/4.5 kg from the buttocks and tummy would be wonderful. If we could confine our fat reduction to specific areas such as our buttocks or our waist area a loss of 10 lb/4.5 kg may be significant, but unfortunately the weight loss process does not work this way. The process of losing fat is a mirrored reversal of the fat gaining procedure and involves all of the fat on our bodies and not just the areas we would like to see reduced.

A WEIGHT LOSS PROGRAM FOR CHILDREN

One in every three children in Australia is suffering from the condition of being overweight or obesity, yet radical dieting is not usually necessary. Most children respond favourably to modest changes in their diet and activity levels. Breakfast should consist of protein such as scrambled egg or an omelette, or perhaps a meat product with or without egg. Carbohydrate intake should be restricted and limited to just one slice of toast with butter. Jam, jelly and sweetened peanut butter and sauces should be avoided. Breakfast cereals are high in natural sugar and should also be avoided, especially sugar-added breakfast cereals such as Coco Pops and Frosties. Restrict bread intake at lunch to two slices and include protein such as chicken or other cold meat, and perhaps some carrot or celery sticks. Dinner should include protein and at least two vegetables including a yellow and a green vegetable. Choose high fibre and nutrient rich vegetables such as carrots, pumpkin, squash, spinach, beans and broccoli. A small serve of potato is acceptable. Restrict fruit intake to two pieces each day and milk to one glass at each meal. Eliminate cake, cookies, candy, chocolate and dried fruit from the diet, and restrict ice-cream consumption to a small serve twice weekly in place of one piece of fruit.

Snacks should be savoury such as crackers with cheese or other protein, or perhaps carrot and celery sticks. As all children are in a rapid growth phase allow them to eat as much as they want at the dinner table, but after meal snacks, especially those containing sugar, should be avoided.

As additional body fat is often synonymous with inactivity, you should encourage your child to sit less and play more. As a child's activity level increases and the amount of excess body fat decreases, less parental encouragement will be required.

WEIGHT LOSS FOR TEENAGERS

For those readers who have not yet reached their twentieth year of life, assess what you consider your lean body weight should be for your current age and body type and use that as your starting point. But please be honest with yourself. If you have a large frame or a naturally robust build do not downgrade your weight to that of your favourite film star or sporting hero. We cannot change our genetic body types, but we can change how we look and how we feel, given what we have.

If you are in your early to mid-teens and still growing, your lean body weight will continue to increase naturally until you reach full maturity. Bone growth ceases at about the seventeenth year of life, but muscle and soft tissue continue to develop for another two or three years. As your optimum daily food intake allowances are directly governed by your lean body weight it is imperative you reassess your program every five months during this growth period and recalculate your food intake levels accordingly. Natural body growth must be taken into consideration in order to maintain optimum health and body development.

CALCULATING YOUR DAILY FOOD ALLOWANCE

Tables 1.1 and 1.2 are quick reference charts presented in both
the imperial and metric measuring systems. By choosing the
table best suited to your purpose you may quickly calculate your
optimum daily protein and carbohydrate intake levels. To
further simplify the process, two fill-in-the-blank personal assessment exercises appear at the bottom of each table. These will
enable you to record your **during weight loss** and **during weight
maintenance** daily protein and carbohydrate allowances.

If you choose the imperial chart you will notice the daily
protein allowance is given in ounces but the daily carbohydrate
allowance is given in grams. There is good reason for this.
The most nutritional foods are those at the bottom of the
carbohydrate content scale and most contain sugar in amounts
not easily calculated in ounces. For example, a large serving of
green beans contains one gram of carbohydrate, the equivalent
of just ⅟₂₈ th part of an ounce. As the use of fractions would
make your task extremely difficult, the simpler international
standard of grams has been retained. You may find it easier to
think of your food as containing units of sugar and not grams of
sugar. For example, if your daily carbohydrate allowance is
40 gm, think of this number as being 40 units of carbohydrate
and there will be no confusion.

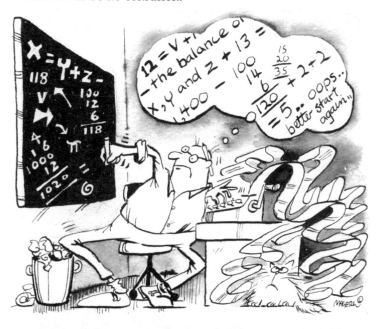

LEAN BODY WEIGHT	DAILY PROTEIN ALLOWANCE	DAILY CARBOHYDRATE ALLOWANCE (wt loss)	DAILY CARBOHYDRATE ALLOWANCE (wt maintenance)
▼1	▼2	▼3	▼4
(in pounds)	(in ounces)	(in grams)	(in grams)
86–90	9	23	34
91–95	9.5	24	36
96–100	10	25	38
101–105	10.5	27	40
106–110	11	28	42
111–115	11.5	29	44
116–120	12	31	46
121–125	12.5	32	48
126–130	13	33	49
131–135	13.5	34	51
136–140	14	35	53
141–145	14.5	37	55
146–150	15	38	57
151–155	15.5	39	59
156–160	16	41	61
161–165	16.5	42	63
166–170	17	43	65
171–175	17.5	44	66
176–180	18	46	68
181–185	18.5	47	70
186–190	19	48	72
191–195	19.5	49	74
196–200	20	51	76
201–205	20.5	52	78

For each 5 lb or part thereof over 205 lb lean body weight add
.5 oz   1 g   2 g

Your personalised daily food intake assessment

During weight loss

Protein........................oz

Carbohydrate.............g

During weight maintenance

Protein........................oz

Carbohydrate.............g

Protein and Carbohydrate Assessment Chart
Imperial Measuring System

Table 1.1

LEAN BODY WEIGHT ▼1 (in kilograms)	DAILY PROTEIN ALLOWANCE ▼2 (in grams)	DAILY CARBOHYDRATE ALLOWANCE (wt loss) ▼3 (in grams)	DAILY CARBOHYDRATE ALLOWANCE (wt maintenance) ▼4 (in grams)
37–39	245	22	33
40–42	265	24	35
43–45	280	25	38
46–48	300	27	40
49–51	320	29	43
52–54	340	30	45
55–57	360	32	48
58–60	375	34	50
61–63	395	35	53
64–66	415	37	55
67–69	435	39	58
70–72	450	40	60
73–75	470	42	63
76–78	490	43	65
79–81	510	45	67
82–84	525	47	70
85–87	545	49	73
88–90	565	50	75
91–93	580	52	78
94–96	600	54	80

For each 1 kg or part thereof over 96 kg lean body weight add

	5g	.5g	1g

Your personalised daily food intake assessment

During weight loss

Protein.......................g

Carbohydrate.............g

During weight maintenance

Protein........................g

Carbohydrate.............g

Protein and Carbohydrate Assessment Chart
Metric Measuring System

Table 1.2

You can readily calculate your optimum daily food intake allowance for both the **during weight loss** and **during weight maintenance** parts of your program by following these four very simple steps.

STEP 1   *Determining your weight range*

Look down column 1 and select the range of weights containing your lean body weight. For example, if you choose the imperial option and your lean body weight is 114 lb you would select the 111–115 lb range. Alternatively, if you choose the metric option and your lean body weight is 52 kg, you would choose the 52–54 kg range.

STEP 2   *Determining your daily protein allowance*

Your protein allowance will remain constant during both parts of your program, so record the figure appearing in column 2 opposite your weight range in the spaces marked *protein* in both the **during weight loss** and **during weight maintenance** assessments.

STEP 3   *Determining your daily 'during weight loss' carbohydrate allowance*

On the same line as your range of weights, record the value appearing in column 3 in the space marked *carbohydrate* in the **during weight loss** assessment.

STEP 4   *Determining your 'during weight maintenance' daily carbohydrate allowance*

On the same line as your range of weights, record the value appearing in column 4 in the space marked *carbohydrate* in the **during weight maintenance** assessment.

There you have it. Your own personal optimum daily intake allowance for the major food groups of protein and carbohydrate. These values represent a lifetime balance of foods capable of transforming you into a slimmer, healthier and happier person, and keeping you that way *forever*.

Before we move on let us clearly understand what these facts and figures mean.

Proteins

Proteins are the muscle and tissue building foods and include all of the food sources listed in Table 1.3.

Bacon	Fish, all types	Pork, all cuts
Beef, all cuts	Game, all types	Prawns
Cheese	Lamb, all cuts	Scallops
Chicken	Lobster	Shrimp
Crab	Mussels	Turkey
Duck	Oysters	Veal
Eggs		

Complete Protein Sources

Table 1.3

Your optimum daily protein allowance refers to the *uncooked weight of the protein source itself*. For example, if your daily protein allowance is 16 oz/450 g you may eat any combination of protein food you choose, provided the combined weight of the chosen food does not exceed your total daily allowance of 16 oz/450 g. Eggs are an exception to the total protein rule. An egg comes packaged in a shell, which of course you will not eat. As a rule of thumb, the protein content of an egg is approximately half the weight of the whole egg, including the shell.

Cheese is measured in its natural state, but reduce your protein allowance by 15% if you are weighing any product listed in Table 1.3 after it has been cooked.

Some vegetables, nuts and grains contain traces of protein but in such small quantities as to be irrelevant. Your *Slim Forever* assessment process has been designed for simp-licity so disregard the protein content of all food other than that contained in the complete protein food sources listed in Table 1.3.

Carbohydrates

Carbohydrates are the food sources which contain natural or added sugar. Commonly referred to as the energy source foods they are also the foods which are most fattening. The major carbohydrate food groups are listed in Table 1.4.

Beer	Fruit, dried	Pasta
Biscuits	Fruit, fresh	Pies and pasties
Bread	Fruit juice	Puddings
Breakfast cereals	Grains	Salad dressings
Cake	Honey	Soft drinks
Candy	Ice-cream	Spirits
Chocolate	Jams and jellies	Sugar
Cookies	Ketchup and sauces	Vegetables
Crackers	Milk, fat reduced	Wine
Cream	Milk, whole	Yoghurt

Carbohydrate Food Sources

Table 1.4

Do not be alarmed. You may still eat and drink from this list but you must do so in moderation. Carbohydrate in our diet is absolutely essential to the life process, but if consumed to excess it will lock you into fat formation and inhibit fat release for energy.

Carbohydrate is sugar in all of its many forms, but unlike protein which is measured by the actual weight of the food itself, carbohydrate is measured not by the weight of the food but by the *amount of sugar each particular food contains*. For example, some vegetables in their natural state contain less than 1% carbohydrate, but refined cane sugar (a substance added liberally to almost all processed foods) is 100% pure carbohydrate.

In calculating your daily carbohydrate intake allowance please remember it is not the bulk of the food source that is of concern, but rather the amount of natural or added sugar each particular food contains. To enable you to easily calculate just how much carbohydrate is present in a particular food, a detailed *Carbohydrate counter* is presented in Part III. It lists most foods in alphabetical order, and in groups according to the relative fat forming potential of each particular food.

Unlike most diets which restrict you to a narrow range of often tasteless and boring foods, there are no menu restrictions with the *Slim Forever* program. The choice of food is yours provided always the sum of your consumed proteins and carbohydrates is not greater, or less, than your optimum daily allowances.

Protein from animal sources remains relatively constant irrespective of the source, but the amount of carbohydrate in sugar bearing foods varies considerably between food sources. Therefore, the lower the carbohydrate content of a particular food, the more you can eat of that food either singularly or in combination with other carbohydrate foods.

The secret to success is to balance your intake of carbohydrate foods so you get plenty to eat, and so avoid feeling hungry. For example, 3.5 oz/100 g by weight of fresh asparagus contains just 1 g of carbohydrate, but 3.5 oz/100 g by weight of Rice Bubbles or Rice Krispies contains 88 g of carbohydrate. If your optimum daily carbohydrate allowance is 44 g, you could, if you wish, eat 10 lb/4.4 kg of asparagus, but only 2 oz/50 g of some breakfast cereals before exhausting your total daily carbohydrate allowance. It is unlikely you would eat 10 lb/4.4 kg of asparagus in one day but this example does demonstrate the enormous differences in the sugar content of various carbohydrate foods.

Let us look at a more realistic comparison using fruit cake as the villain. A single slice of fruit cake weighing 2 oz/60 g contains approximately 38 g of carbohydrate. Instead of eating the fruit cake you could choose, for example, an appetiser of 3.5 oz/100 g by weight of avocado vinaigrette (2); followed by a main course of protein such as red meat, fish or poultry, together with 3.5 oz/100 g by weight of French beans (1); 3.5 oz/100 g by weight of cauliflower (1); 3.5 oz/100 g by weight of boiled new potatoes (18) and 3.5 oz/100 g by weight of fresh strawberries (9). You may also choose a glass of wine or other beverage of similar sugar content (6) and you could put a little butter on your beans (0), cheese sauce on your cauliflower (.5), cream on your strawberries (.5) and lose weight while you were eating. The bracketed figures appearing after each suggested food source represent the amount of carbohydrate it contains. In this example the total is 38 g the equal of a small slice of fruit cake.

Again using the above example, you could forego the beverage if you wished, and use the additional 6 g of carbohydrate by choosing extra fruit or vegetables. Or, you may choose to replace the suggested carbohydrate foods with foods of higher carbohydrate content such as a small serve of pasta or ice-cream. All of these options are available to you provided the sum of your carbohydrate foods does not exceed your optimum daily allowance.

Your body does not concern itself with the source of the protein or carbohydrate you consume. Protein from red meat is the same as protein from white meat, and carbohydrate from fruit and vegetables is the same as carbohydrate from a chocolate cookie. You could eat your daily allowance of protein together with a small slice of fruit cake and still lose weight provided you don't eat anything else, but, you would be hungry and very soon unhealthy. For the sake of your appetite and your health choose carbohydrates that are both filling and nutritious.

As always there is the exception. Mushrooms are a vegetable moderately high in vitamins and minerals but they are carbohydrate and protein free. You may eat as many mushrooms as you please at any time of the day or night, even during **weight loss**.

Fats and oils

Fresh fats and oils are as important to your diet and good health as are the proteins and carbohydrates, but they too must be consumed in moderation. Any food eaten to excess, including fats and oils, will form unwanted body fat. So, limit your fat intake by removing all but $\frac{1}{8}$ in/3 mm of fat from precooked meat and skim any excess fat from braises, stews and curries. Use butter sparingly and eliminate margarine from your diet.

Olive and peanut oils are classified as being mono-unsaturated, and are by far the healthiest and the best of the readily available oils for salad dressings and for cooking, but use them sparingly.

A balanced daily intake of vitamins, minerals and dietary bulk is also of major importance, and these subjects are covered in detail in Part II. As a general guide to carbohydrate intake, choose either a fresh garden salad or two or three cooked vegetables and perhaps a piece of fruit to accompany your evening meal. Contrary to popular belief, your body does not require a mountain of vitamins and minerals to function. By varying your diet to include a cross-section of green and yellow vegetables and some fruit, you will supply your body with all the vitamins, minerals and dietary bulk essential for good health.

It may appear at first glance that you will be spending the rest of your life weighing and calculating the sugar content of the foods you eat, but this is not so in practice. You will need to weigh and keep track of what you are eating and drinking for a few days. However, you will soon learn how much of a particular food you can eat and in what combinations. This is a lifelong commitment to being slimmer, healthier and living longer, and the effort involved for a few days of weighing and experimenting will be well rewarded.

To assist you in getting to know just how adventurous you can be in selecting and planning meals, Part III of this book is devoted to some simple recipes and suggested meal combinations you will surely find exciting.

The *Slim Forever* program is a blueprint of healthy eating, so be imaginative and please don't treat it as a diet. And above all, avoid mealtime boredom. If you desire a food higher in carbohydrate, eat a smaller quantity of that food and compliment it with foods low in carbohydrate and you will not feel deprived.

The only claim to fame many diets are able to make is their success in alienating you from your family and your friends, but not so your *Slim Forever* program. Eating is a very pleasurable experience which has become something of a ritual in our modern day society. Family get-togethers, dinner parties and social functions need no longer be removed from your calendar just because you are reducing your body weight. You may continue to be social, and to satisfy your hunger and your palate with filling, tasty and nutritionally balanced meals, just by following a few very simple rules. By balancing your intake of the various food groups you need never feel hungry again, and you need never reasonably forego any of your favourite foods, or become a social outcast.

Bon appétit!

2 the golden rules of being slim forever

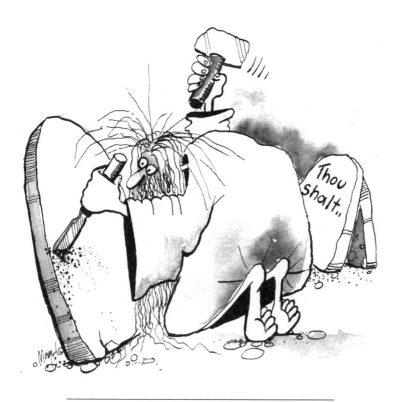

Ten simple steps to healthy living

The *Slim Forever* program is really very simple to understand and to follow, and your participation will cost no more than the price of this book. You will not be required to attend meetings, to eat tasteless or boring food, or to ever feel hungry again. You can follow this program at home, at work, or at play, provided you adhere to these very simple rules.

TEN SIMPLE STEPS TO HEALTHY LIVING

RULE 1   *Do not eat more or less protein or carbohydrate than is indicated by your personal daily intake allowances*

Of these two groups, the amount of carbohydrate you consume is the most critical. Too little carbohydrate will dangerously lower your blood sugar levels, and too much will stop you from losing unwanted body fat.

Low levels of protein intake will result in muscle and tissue wasting, and may endanger your long-term health, but excessive protein consumption may result in the unused portion being converted into body fat.

RULE 2   *Do not eat less protein or carbohydrate today because you want to eat more tomorrow*

Your body operates in strict accordance with the dictates of its very own 24-hour biological clock as explained in Chapter 18. All body reactions are absolute, and any dietary excess or deficiency will be accepted for what it is, and on the day it occurs. There is no time off for good behaviour.

RULE 3   *Do not consume any carbohydrate prior to your evening meal during weight loss*

This is perhaps the most important of all the rules and forms the basis of the *Slim Forever* program.

During **weight loss**, any carbohydrate consumed during the day (and this includes toast for breakfast, cereal, fruit, vegetables, fruit juices, soft drinks etc) will abort the fat burning process. Eat all of your allowable carbohydrate with, or soon after your evening meal.

Do not be alarmed. It is only in recent years that we have forsaken a cooked breakfast in favour of cereal and toast, much to the detriment of our overall health. The food choices available to you for both breakfast and lunch are almost limitless. Part III presents just some of these filling and appetite suppressing foods which you will surely enjoy.

Once you move to **weight maintenance** your optimum daily carbohydrate intake allowance will increase by 50%. As you will no longer be seeking to actively burn body fat, you may now eat these sugar containing foods at any time of the day or evening, and still maintain your weight. You may, if you wish, resume eating toast and fruit for breakfast and a salad for lunch, provided the sum of the carbohydrate foods you consume during the entire day does not exceed your new optimum daily intake allowance.

Protein is the exception. You can eat protein at any time of the day or evening during **weight loss** and during **weight maintenance**, provided the total weight of the protein you eat does not exceed your optimum daily allowance. During **weight loss** your breakfast and lunch will have to consist entirely of protein as the presence of additional sugar in your system during the day will abort the fat burning process.

Limit your protein intake during the day to a maximum of 50% of your total daily allowance, and consume at least 50% of your protein with your evening meal.

RULE 4   *Include some fresh oils and fats in your daily diet*

Fresh fats, as opposed to damaged processed fats, are essential for good health and well-being. Dietary fat is necessary for the manufacture within our bodies of life-giving prostaglandins, to build resistance to disease, and to inhibit excess fat formation. Leave a little fat on your meat, eat butter not margarine, and where possible use olive and peanut oils for cooking and salad dressings.

Saturated fats are not the villains they were thought to be in the elevated blood cholesterol debate. The exclusion of fats from the diet is a clinically proven precursor to many health problems, not the least of which are insatiable hunger and uncontrollable weight gain. These subjects are addressed in detail in Part II.

RULE 5 *Occasional overindulgence is not a mortal sin*

It is unlikely you will reach your desired weight without overindulging yourself at least once, but do not despair. To err is to be human.

Any interruption to your **weight loss** program will not result in you suddenly gaining unwanted body fat, unless your binge is outrageous and lasts for days. If you do interrupt your program, it will take from one to three days, depending upon the magnitude of your binge, to lower your blood sugar level sufficiently for the fat burning process to reactivate. Once reactivated, it will be another three or four days before your body again reaches maximum fat burning potential.

Please remember, your body cannot burn stored body fat as energy in any quantity if there is excessive sugar in your blood stream. The fat burning process will only fully reactivate when your blood sugar level is significantly reduced, at which point your body will burn predominantly fat and very little glucose for the production of energy.

If you do binge you can accelerate a reduction in your blood sugar levels by reducing your daily carbohydrate intake by 30% for one day following a minor binge; for two days following a significant binge; and for three days following a total pig out. Under no circumstances reduce your carbohydrate intake for longer than three days, or your blood sugar will fall below a controllable level. Drastically reduced blood sugar levels signal starvation and your body will switch from converting stored fat, to converting essential muscle and very little fat for the production of energy.

A short-term binge is not measured in fat gain but in time lost in achieving your long-term goal. If you do interrupt your program make sure it is for good reason and worth the effort.

Once you enter **weight maintenance** this method of accelerated blood sugar reduction will help you burn your excess blood sugar before it can be converted to stored body fat. However, as you will no longer be in the weight loss mode, you will not suffer the time loss associated with overeating.

Your body can cope with the occasional binge, but a pattern of constantly alternating between binges and periods of reduced carbohydrate consumption will take its toll on your health. Practise moderation in all things and you and your body will be pals for a long time.

RULE 6   *You are an extension of what you eat*

Your body depends entirely on the foods you eat for its supply of energy and for the ongoing process of building tissue. Conversely, your body has no option other than to accept what you eat, and process it, irrespective of the consequences. A body fed rubbish cannot be expected to perform as well as a body fed a balanced and nutritional diet of energy and body building foods. Your body is where you live so be sensible with your food choices.

If you treat your body with the same respect most of us seem to have for our cars you can look forward to a long and healthy life. Abuse either one and it will soon break down.

RULE 7   *Do not follow another person's customised daily carbohydrate and protein allowances*

A **weight loss** program not tailored to your specific lean body weight is potentially ineffective, and may even be dangerous. Protect your health by assessing your own optimum daily food allowance using the *Slim Forever* formula.

RULE 8   *Trouble shooting your failure to lose stored body fat*

Recent studies conducted by the Commonwealth Scientific and Industrial Research Organisation (CSIRO) in Australia have raised doubt over the issue of overweight people having slower basal metabolic rates (the rate at which a body burns energy) than do slimmer people. Tests indicate that basal metabolic rates between individuals do not alter upwards or downwards by greater than 7.5%. The same tests do, however, indicate that females have a greater predilection to changes in metabolic rate than males.

There is no evidence yet at hand to indicate differences in the absorption rates of nutrients between individuals, but it cannot be denied that certain individuals appear to have a greater propensity for gaining weight. This may be linked to each person's relative ability to mobilise stored body fat for energy, but, whatever the reason, you may have to reduce your overall food intake if you are not losing body fat.

If you fail to reduce your level of excess body fat you have probably violated one or more of the following criteria:

1 you may have miscalculated your base body weight;

2 you may be consuming more than your optimum daily allowances of either carbohydrate or protein, or both; or

3 you may have an ultra-efficient nutrient absorption system.

If you have faithfully followed your *Slim Forever* program for two weeks and you have failed to lose weight, simply go up one line on the *Protein and carbohydrate assessment charts* (Tables 1.1 and 1.2) and use the lesser values for both protein and carbohydrate intake. If after an additional two weeks you still fail to lose weight, go one line higher again.

Seldom has any person in trials so far conducted had to reduce their protein and carbohydrate intake more than once, and certainly no one to date has had to reduce these levels more than twice. If your failure to lose weight continues, you have probably made a gross error in calculating your lean body weight, or your optimum food intake allowances, or both.

RULE 9 *Don't count calories*

Calories, and their metric counterpart kilojoules, are a measure of the energy content of food. The validity of the calorie and kilojoule theory is highly questionable and is dealt with in detail in Chapter 6.

Restrict your calculations to the protein and carbohydrate content of the foods you eat as outlined in the *Slim Forever* program.

RULE 10 *Don't be impatient*

The *Slim Forever* program is not a crash diet. It is a balanced and scientifically proven safe weight loss and weight maintenance program. You will lose body fat, and the loss will be safe and sustainable, but it will take time. Remember, this is a lifelong commitment to being slimmer and healthier, and you will reach your goal very quickly, so be a little patient. It will be worth every ounce of effort expended.

If you find the going restrictive, you can take a break from **weight loss** by moving to **weight maintenance** for a short period. However, you must stay on **weight loss** for at least 21 days for it to be effective.

Some people have the ability to apply themselves to a task and not draw breath until it is completed, while others need interim goals. If you choose to take a break it will take longer to reach your goal. But, if time is what you have and you feel you need to take a break, this routine may well work best for you.

This rule can also be applied to vacations and festive events such as special dinners, birthdays, Christmas and Thanksgiving should they fall during the **weight loss** part of your program. There is absolutely no reason for you to feel left out, provided you are sensible and you follow these very simple rules.

monitoring your progress

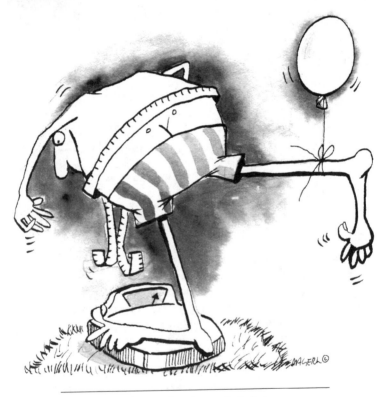

Carbohydrate intake

Changes in body function

Your expectations

Rate of fat reduction

Weight maintenance

Being overweight or obese does not necessarily imply gluttony. Controlling your weight is not so much a matter of monitoring how much food you eat, but rather, what you eat. You can gain weight by eating an overabundance of healthy foods just as surely as you can gain weight from eating sugary junk. Many overweight people eat surprisingly small meals and still fail to lose unwanted body fat, or even worse, they continue to gain weight. This fact was clearly demonstrated by a number of participants in the *Slim Forever* control groups who, during the first two weeks, complained of having difficulty in eating all of the food necessary to reach their optimum food intake levels. They persisted, and as their bodies adjusted to a totally balanced diet, they shed body fat, yet they were eating more food than they had previously.

Nothing can be achieved without a little effort, and the process of losing excess body fat and keeping it off is no exception. To achieve the very best results from your *Slim Forever* program, and in the shortest possible time, you will need to apply yourself to the task. The **weight loss** part of your program is the most critical and will demand your closest attention. Old habits die hard, but old in this case does not necessarily imply good. For better or for worse much of our daily eating is dominated by habit, and the breaking of any habit will create short-term confusion in our minds and in our bodies. But, change we must if we want to achieve our goals.

CARBOHYDRATE INTAKE

Not eating carbohydrate during the day while you are actively in **weight loss** will probably be the most difficult change you will be required to make. Surprisingly, the things you feel you cannot do without today will not have the same significance in another week or so. The revelation that no carbohydrate could be consumed prior to the evening meal during **weight loss** was met by groans of disapproval from members of the control groups. The protesters were especially vocal about no toast for breakfast. Almost without exception, and within just two weeks of commencing the program, these same people confessed they no longer missed, nor even desired, the foods they thought they could not do without – and this included their traditional breakfast toast. You may if you wish resume eating carbohydrate during the day, including toast for breakfast, once you reach the **weight maintenance** part of your program. But, under no circumstances may you do this during **weight loss**.

The eradication of carbohydrate foods from your diet during the day is necessary during **weight loss** if you are to break down the excess fat deposits in your body. In order to lose body fat you must induce your body to switch from burning predominantly blood sugar, to burning stored fat as its immediate energy source. This can only be achieved by specifically lowering your overall intake of carbohydrate foods, which in turn will reduce your blood sugar levels. However, any reduction in carbohydrate intake must be conducted under conditions of absolute control as indicated by your optimum daily intake allowance.

The human body will sense starvation after just two or three days of food deprivation. The basis of the *Slim Forever* program was the discovery that the effective long-term burning of body fat for energy in sufficient quantities to effect meaningful body fat loss can only be sustained initially for a maximum of five to six hours each day. Any period of prolonged fat loss beyond this limit will cause your body to sense starvation and to commence breaking down muscle in favour of stored body fat.

By specifically controlling carbohydrate intake you can maximise body fat loss without signalling starvation. The carbohydrate you consume with your evening meal will supply your body with sufficient blood sugar to last until early afternoon the following day. During this period your body will register normal sugar burning function, together with some stored fat. When your immediate supply of blood sugar becomes sufficiently reduced your body will switch to burning predominantly stored fat for energy. When the carbohydrate from your next evening meal enters your blood stream, fat loss will cease, and the 24 hour process, including five to six hours of fat loss, will be repeated.

CHANGES IN BODY FUNCTION

The switch from burning predominantly sugar to burning predominantly fat for energy will probably be a new experience for you. Although the mechanism for change is inherently in place, it is likely there will be a period of hesitation between the end of the sugar burning process and the commencement of the fat burning process. Our bodies function according to a complicated and integrated system of primary and secondary controls and learned responses, but some of these responses have to be re-programmed. Preparation for the switch in emphasis from blood sugar to stored fat for the production of energy will commence well before your level of blood sugar is depleted. As this is not yet a practised response, short-term hesitation in achieving the switch may lead to a mild state of low blood sugar, or induced hypoglycaemia. Should this occur you may experience the onset of sudden tiredness, irritability, and bad breath, but, as soon as the switch to burning stored fat is complete, the symptoms will abate. Uncontrolled hypoglycaemia associated with organ dysfunction or starvation can be dangerous, but with the *Slim Forever* program this mild hypoglycaemic state will be minimal, totally controlled, and absolutely safe. After a few days the switch from burning mostly glucose to burning mostly fat for the production of energy will take place without hesitation and any discomfort you may have previously felt will cease.

The change in the balance of foods you consume may initiate changes in your bowel function. Reactions vary between individuals, with some reporting no apparent change at all, while others experience the onset of either loose stools or constipation. In a few cases, the onset of loose stools may be followed by constipation.

The intake of a balanced diet will initiate a cleansing of the bowel of any faecal deposits associated with past imbalances in food intake. Overeating often results in chunks of impacted faeces forming in the colon, which can in time grow to obstruct the free passage of bowel contents. The evacuated faeces due to bowel cleansing may have an unpleasant odour, and may appear very dark or almost black and tar-like in colour and consistency. This is the result of prolonged enzymatic and bacterial action on the faeces as it lay dormant in the bowel. If this should occur, do not be alarmed. Your body is simply seizing the opportunity to rid itself of a pest, and the process usually only takes a day or two.

Constipation may occur for one of two reasons. The fluids in the foods you eat and drink are absorbed mostly in the small intestine, but the final control over the fluid consistency of faecal material is undertaken in the bowel. If you drink too little fluid, or if too much fluid is drawn off in the bowel, the faeces will be dry and constipation will occur. Our bodies require a constant supply of fluids, preferably water, to survive. Fruit and vegetables contain a high percentage of water, not to mention soft drinks, beer, and copious cups of coffee, the liquid mainstays of many unbalanced diets. On the other hand, protein has a low fluid content, and therefore needs to be consumed along with additional fluids.

The greater part of the human body is water, yet few of us drink water on a daily basis. Over the years we have come to rely on the fluid content of manufactured and often sugar-laden drinks to satisfy our needs. As the intake of these harmful and fat-forming drinks must be reduced during **weight loss**, some participants in the program forget to drink anything at all, and they become constipated. Give your body the fluid it needs by drinking at least four or five glasses of cool fresh water each day. In most cases, the problem of constipation will be overcome.

Chronic constipation may also occur when the bowel becomes obstructed by large chunks of impacted faecal material, or when the motility of the bowel is lost. In the first instance, a course of natural laxative obtained from your health food store at a dose rate of once every three days until the bowel is cleared will usually solve the problem. Bowel motility, or the ability of the bowel to rhythmically contract to move the faecal material along its length, is usually associated with diminished nerve supply to the muscles of the bowel. As the nerves to the bowel exit the spinal cord just above the level of the hips, a tendency to suffer from low back pain often accompanies chronic constipation. If this fits your profile and your constipation persists, you may consider seeking the opinion of a chiropractor.

YOUR EXPECTATIONS

Once you have embarked on your **weight loss** program it will take from three to five days for your body to burn off the excess sugar in your blood and for the fat burning process to commence. Once under way it will take another three or four days to reach full fat burning potential, a potential proportionate to the sum of your lean body weight and your daily activity level.

Stored body fat is not the inert mass it was once thought to be. A small percentage of your stored body fat is in a constant state of movement from the fat storage cells and into the blood stream. If energy-ready fat in the blood stream is not used in the production of energy, these fat molecules will be reabsorbed back into the fat storage cells, and the process repeated. This constant mobilisation of stored fat keeps a supply of readily available fat molecules, or *triglycerides* as they are properly termed, in the blood stream for the production of energy at the cellular level. Once your body switches to burning the available energy-ready triglycerides, the release of additional fat from within the storage cells will increase in proportion to your energy demand, and the fat reduction process will be under way.

RATE OF FAT REDUCTION

The approximate rate of fat reduction you can expect each week during **weight loss** is determined by two factors:

1 your lean body weight; and

2 your physical activity level.

Of these two factors your lean body weight will be the most important. A smaller body will use proportionately less energy than a larger body under similar physical load. However, the undertaking of normal activities without additional exercise will usually result in a sustained fat loss of between 1 lb 12 oz/800 g and 2 lb 3 oz/1 kg each week.

The demonstrated failure of diets to reduce excess levels of body fat has lead to the erroneous conclusion that dieting without exercise will not work. Not so. Most diets fail simply because they lack the ability to induce the body to mobilise stored fat for energy. Tests involving the *Slim Forever* program indicate that even intense physical activity will not increase a person's ability to lose excess body fat by greater than 15% over losses experienced under normal physical activity.

Your early weight loss may not be fat

Your apparent weight loss during the first two weeks will be confusing as it normally includes the loss of excess body fluids and a reduction in the amount of retained faecal material in your bowel. As stored body fat retains large quantities of water, you will shed somewhere between 2 lb/1 kg and 8 lb/4 kg of excess fluid during the first month, together with a reasonable amount of body fat. It is this loss of excess body fluid that many people on starvation diet programs confuse with fat loss.

If by the end of your second week you fail to register a weight loss at least equal to that predicted on page 31, you may be the proud owner of a very efficient gastrointestinal absorption system. Or, more probably, you will have made an error in calculating either your lean body weight or your daily food allowance, or both. Should this occur the problem can be rectified by following the instructions outlined in Rule 8 of *The golden rules of being slim forever*.

Dealing with a weight loss plateau

One in three people exhibit a sharp reduction in fat loss after about three months of sustained loss. This is caused by a shift in emphasis from burning glucose to burning stored fat in the production of body energy. As less carbohydrate is now required for the production of energy and, as the body is now producing glucose from fat, what was previously your optimum daily intake may now be excessive. To overcome a plateau, simply retain your present intake of protein and reduce your carbohydrate intake one line on the *Protein and carbohydrate assessment chart*. If you do not return to your previous rate of weight loss after two weeks, repeat the process and reduce your carbohydrate intake one more line. It should not be necessary to reduce your carbohydrate intake more than twice.

Once you reach the weight maintenance portion of your program you will have to recalculate your daily carbohydrate intake allowance. As your need for carbohydrate has reduced, your weight maintenance carbohydrate level will be calculated based on your reduced weight loss carbohydrate intake allowance, not your original carbohydrate allowance. Simply record the weight maintenance carbohydrate allowance appearing in column 4 on the same line as your new weight loss carbohydrate allowance. And remember, you must maintain your original protein allowance.

How to monitor your progress

Your bathroom scale will be a guide to your progress, but do not rely on it to accurately indicate your net fat loss. The loss of excess body fluids and faecal material has to be considered, and as many of us are protein deficient, there is a high probability you will undergo some increase in muscle density. Do not fear ladies, you will not develop bulging muscles unless you involve yourself in heavy resistance exercise, but you will develop a pleasing level of functional muscle tone.

You may better rationalise your progress by combining the measuring of your thighs, waist, chest and arms with a weekly check of your weight on your bathroom scale, and be guided by how you look in the mirror and how your clothes fit. Even though your progressive recorded weight chart may not be an absolute indication of your net fat loss, be assured there will be no doubt in your mind as to your progress.

Body fat comes off almost as it went on, but in reverse. Fat storage cells are distributed over most of the surface of the human body between the skin and outer muscle layers. Fat cells, with an elastic outer casement of protein of almost infinite stretchability, usually contain at least a small deposit of stored fat, even in the very slim. With nowhere else to go, almost everything you eat in excess of your daily nutrient requirement will be converted into fat, and these trillions of omnipresent fat storage cells will each receive a share of the spoils. Once the fat storage cells around your waist, buttocks and thighs reach a certain level of fat engorgement, adjacent fat storage cells will start to fill. A constant bombardment of triglycerides will create a pyramid effect with the early cells continuing to engorge themselves, while more and more peripheral cells are forced into action.

By controlling both the quantity and quality of the foods you eat during **weight loss**, your body will be forced to switch from burning predominantly blood glucose to burning predominantly stored fat as its major energy source. This controlled process will enable you to safely lose your stores of unwanted body fat without sacrificing essential muscle for the production of energy, as is the case with most starvation diets. Once initiated, the fat burning process will call on all of your fat storage cells to contribute a portion of their energy-ready contents, and quantitative loss will be directly proportional to the amount of fat each cell contains. As the greater proportion of fat is carried around the waist, buttocks and thighs these will be the last cells to empty.

We tend to be an impatient lot, and it is in our nature to want everything to happen today and in a way we would like. Fat reduction from the most obvious areas may not occur as fast as you wish, but it is happening in accordance with the dictates of our unalterable biological structure. A point to remember is, a fat cell under siege to give up its contents will reduce in density long before it reduces in size. This phenomenon may have you believing either that you are not losing weight in the areas important to you, or, that you are actually getting flabbier. A reduction in fat density will reduce much of the bulk of the fat cell well before the outer membrane of the cell itself starts to shrink, but given time, shrink it will. Be patient. Your excess of stored fat will be coming off thirty or forty times faster than it went on, and as the emptying cells begin to shrink, the apparent flabby look will disappear.

The gender factor

Unlike their male counterparts, women form fat on their buttocks and thighs with an 'orange peel' appearance. Although this fat formation is often referred to as cellulite, the term is not scientifically validated. It is not clear why the superficial appearance of this fat differs, but appearances aside, it is still fat. Due to the inadequacy of most diets to remove fat from the body, it has become fashionable to suggest cellulite is difficult to lose, but this is not the case. The first apparent site of fat loss with the *Slim Forever* program is the thighs, and this applies to both females and males alike. The unflattering orange peel presentation associated with cellulite will disappear just as soon as the fat itself disappears.

WEIGHT MAINTENANCE

Once you reach your desired level of weight loss you may then move to the **weight maintenance** part of your program. As you will no longer be seeking to lose excess body fat you may now increase your daily carbohydrate intake by 50%. This increase in allowable carbohydrate intake will permit you to reasonably indulge even more of your food fantasies, provided you do so in moderation and in balance with other healthy carbohydrate foods of lower sugar content. You may now eat your daily allowance of carbohydrate at any time during the day or night, and include toast, fruit, or cereal with your breakfast if you so desire. Your body will even tolerate a little overindulgence, provided you do so in moderation and follow *The golden rules of being slim forever*. If you are sensible you will be free to enjoy any food you choose and never again suffer the consequences of gaining unwanted body fat.

Planning ahead

Forward thinking will help you cope with your social activities. You will have little latitude for error during **weight loss**, so your best plan will be to adhere as strictly as you can to your allowable food intake until you reach your goal. If you do overindulge, resume your program the very next day, and although you will inhibit the fat burning process in the short-term, you will certainly not gain weight.

If you have reached your **weight maintenance** goal and you are planning an evening of dining out, restrict or totally eliminate carbohydrate from breakfast and lunch on that day and reduce your carbohydrate intake to your previous **weight loss** level for a day or so after the event. If weekends are the focus of your social activity you may choose to reduce your carbohydrate intake to your previous **weight loss** level for one day before and two days after the weekend. This will allow you to indulge yourself a little more on your chosen days. Even during **weight maintenance** your body will register every gram of carbohydrate you consume. Although you cannot beat the system, by following the rules you can still play the game, and win.

It is important to remember that the *Slim Forever* program has been scientifically developed to complement your natural body design and function. This is not a diet, but rather a lifelong commitment to balancing your food intake, thus allowing you to safely lose unwanted and life-threatening excess body fat and to keep it off *forever*.

The present day problems of being overweight and obesity reasonably indicate that whatever it is we are doing is terribly wrong. Our metabolism has not changed but our diets certainly have, and therein lies the cause of our dilemma.

How our bodies react to the foods we eat is topically discussed in detail in Part II. You may initially consider the content of some of these chapters to be controversial, but the truth usually is. Please take the time to read and understand what has been written. You will find the material interesting, thought provoking and, above all, personally rewarding.

part II

THE WHY

why lose weight?

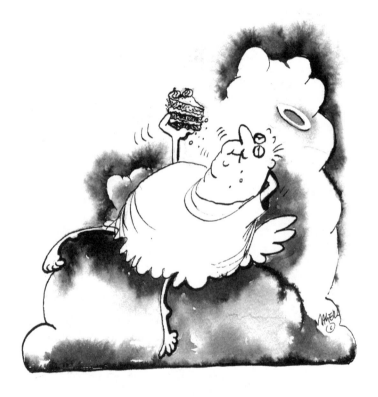

The psychology of being Slim Forever

Is age a barrier to losing weight?

The adverse effects of being overweight (an excess of fat greater than 10% of normal body weight) and obesity (an excess of fat greater than 20% of normal body weight) are staggering. Statistical evidence compiled by life insurance companies suggest a person aged 45 years who is just 10 lb/4.5 kg above normal weight will reduce his or her life span by an estimated 8%. This represents a loss of six years of life for a person who would otherwise have lived to be 75 years old.

Unfortunately the decrease in life expectancy from being overweight or obese is negatively disproportionate to the amount of excess body fat you carry. For example, if a person's excess body fat doubles from 10 lb/4.5 kg to 20 lb/9 kg, the average decrease in longevity will not be 16%, but rather 20%. This represents a frightening reduction in longevity of 15 years from an otherwise possible life span of 75 years.

Simply put, if you are overweight or obese and you don't do something about it, your allotted life span may well be significantly shortened. The imposition of the death sentence just for being overweight indeed appears to be a miscarriage of justice, but our bodies obviously consider the presence of excess body fat to be a far more serious crime than we ourselves consciously admit.

Available figures indicate nine out of every ten people in the United States consider themselves to be overweight. However, the conditions of being overweight and obesity are not confined to the middle and older age groups. Young people too are affected by an overabundance of body fat to an alarming degree. According to the *National Diet Council Report* #2 of 1985, one in every three young Australians is currently classified as being clinically overweight.

Suffering from being overweight and obesity do more than just make us look and feel bad. These monumental problems are costing our societies the needless loss of millions of lives and billions of dollars annually from heart disease, cancer, stroke, diabetes, abdominal herniation, intestinal obstruction, gall bladder disease and stomach ulcers. Professor Zimmet, adviser to the World Health Organization and President of the Australian Society for the Study of Obesity, estimates the treatment of fat-related diseases currently costs the Australian taxpayer $5 billion each year (*Sunday Telegraph*, 19 July 1992). In real terms, for a country with a population of just 17 million people, the money avoidably spent on fat-related diseases is equal to one-third of the current Australian annual national deficit.

What is the alternative?

It has been variously asserted that 60% to 70% of premature deaths from all diseases could be avoided if we as individuals accepted more responsibility for our own health. What has gone wrong? Why, when we have an abundance of food and technical know-how, are we continuing to gain unwanted body fat despite our best efforts to stay slim? And why, after four million years of evolution and relatively slim human existence, do we sud- denly find ourselves besieged by an epidemic of excess body fat?

The answer is simple. Over recent millennia we have imple- mented changes in our dietary habits incompatible with the natural design and function of our bodies. By evolution or creation we are meat eaters, a fact supported by an abundance of scientific, historical and palaeontological evidence. We are clearly the descendants of a race of hunters who supplemented their predominantly red meat diets with nuts and berries foraged from the wild.

Climatic change, the domestication of wild animals and the cultivation of crops altered our eating habits forever. Little by little we increased our intake of fruit, vegetables and sugar laden foods, and correspondingly reduced our intake of meat. As time progressed we learned to create new varieties of fruit and vegetables, and we developed the technology to make them grow larger, in abundance, and in less time.

We have arrived at the crossroads. The complementary meat dominant diets of our natural and evolutionary past have been replaced by diets high in carbohydrate, much to the detriment of our bodies and our health. Long-term survival depends on the ability of a species to live in harmony with its prevailing environmental structure. Or alternatively, it depends on the ability of a species to alter the environment to suit its changing needs. The dinosaurs failed to adapt to changes in their environment and perished, but the highly adaptable prehistoric sharks inhabiting the oceans of this planet continue to thrive despite 300 million years of upheaval and change.

The species *Homo sapiens,* as we are collectively labelled, is not following its dietary destiny. With gathering momentum we are introducing changes which are incompatible with the programmed functions of our highly organised bodies. If we are to survive as individuals, and collectively as a race, we must get back to basics and readopt a diet containing a balance of all the necessary food groups complementary to the natural function and design of our very complex systems.

It has long been said that the inhabitants of the industrialised world are digging their graves with their knives and forks, but never has this statement had greater meaning than it does today. We have innocently created a monster that is striking at the very root of our existence, but we can, with a little understanding and effort, drive the evil fat genie back into the bottle where it belongs.

THE PSYCHOLOGY OF BEING SLIM FOREVER

Recognising the enemy

Considered an advertising genius of his time, Joseph Paul Goebbels was the Minister for Propaganda to Adolf Hitler's Third Reich. He espoused that if you want to tell a lie and have it believed, make it a big lie and tell it often. He wrote 'propaganda has only one objective – to conquer the masses' (*Stars and Stripes,* 1945). Therein lies the philosophy of product advertising in general and of food advertising in particular.

From the moment we accept solid food we become the targets of dietary misinformation and advertising propaganda. To the detriment of the health of entire populations, self-serving food manufacturers advertise their often nutritionally denuded and chemically altered food in an almost utopian fashion.

Food manufacturing and advertising companies employ sociologists and psychologists to seek out and identify any weaknesses the unsuspecting public may have in regard to consuming food. This knowledge is then used to produce television commercials containing both overt and subliminal messages compelling you to buy their product. For example, one of the world's leading cola manufacturers consistently produces commercials depicting very slim and physically attractive young people performing all manner of incredibly athletic feats. Overtly the commercial is selling the product, but subliminally it is suggesting a link between drinking their brand of cola and being slim, physically attractive and incredibly athletic. With 1.4 oz/40 g of sugar, the equivalent of eight teaspoons in every can, perhaps a commercial involving a group of overweight and pimply faced youths standing on a street corner would be more appropriate.

Children are especially targeted and bombarded with immoral television advertising designed to indoctrinate them into the world of sugar addiction. Giving evidence before a United States Senate Select Committee on Nutrition and Human Needs in March 1973, Dr Jean Mayer, the Professor of Nutrition at Harvard School of Public Health, expressed the opinion that the more useless a food product, the greater is its advertising exposure on television. A survey in the United States revealed one 200-minute Saturday morning segment of prime children's television viewing contained 73 advertisements for breakfast cereals, soft drinks, candy, cookies and popcorn. That is an average of one junk food commercial every two minutes and 45 seconds, including the running time of the commercial itself. Another survey, conducted in England, revealed that 41.6% of all advertisements aired during prime children's viewing time promoted chocolate, candy and fast food as compared to 23% during an entire viewing day. With such saturation advertising is it any wonder the youth of the industrialised world are in the grips of a fat explosion.

The enemy of being slim is the junk food manufacturing industry and the advertising stooges who accept their money but none of the guilt for the dishonest commercials they produce. If you are serious about changing the way you look and the way you feel you will have to rise above this multibillion dollar propaganda machine.

Conquering the masses

The nutrition industry itself is not without fault. The linear thinking pattern of an alarming number of professionals, including those involved in health and nutrition, serves to propagate rather than to dispel misinformation. Unscientific postulations which result in the making of recommendations as to how much or how little of a specific food should be consumed are now justifiably being questioned. But, in many cases the damage has already been done.

In a similar manner to the designer clothes industry where fashion takes precedence over practicality, food has been taken out of the arena of nutritional sustenance. We celebrate almost every event, from births to funerals, with food and drink. Business meetings, social gatherings and even the winning of battles and sporting events are not complete unless we indulge ourselves in food. As if eating was not enough, we take the opportunity to stuff ourselves to absolute capacity without guilt. After all, it is a celebration.

We have fashioned food into a weapon which we turn upon ourselves, our family and our friends as often as we possibly can. We use the threat of withholding food to make children behave, or individuals and even entire populations to succumb to tyranny. We also use food as a weapon to induce better effort. Teachers reward children with candy for a job well done which is akin to shooting the winner in the foot. Socially it is considered bad manners not to offer food to visitors, or for a visitor to refuse the food so offered. Often, the more the visitor eats, the greater is considered the hospitality of the host and the appreciation of the visitor. Children are frequently forbidden to leave the table until the food on their plate is gone, not withstanding the choice of food and the portions are that of the parent, not of the child.

Have you ever wondered why so-called friends and associates descend upon a person who is trying to give up smoking, or quit drinking, and prevail upon that person to have a cigarette or a drink? Misery loves company, and it is for this reason many overweight people keep the company of other overweight people. If everyone in the group goes back for seconds at lunch it must be okay, but if just one person refuses, the psychological equilibrium of the group goes out the window. If one member of the group elects to eat a modest lunch, the remainder of the group are openly reminded of just how much they are eating, and that is not acceptable. Rather than the majority of the group modifying their eating habits, it is easier to coerce the maverick member into again eating more.

Boredom and unhappiness are often precursors to overeating. 'Foodaholism' is a disease of no less consequence than alcoholism, but food addiction lacks the metabolic imbalance associated with some alcohol toxicity. Overeating is by way of punishment for low self-esteem, and the results serve as a positive expression of just how worthless the victim really is. In the face of adversity smokers reach for a cigarette, drinkers reach for a bottle and eaters reach for the refrigerator. If this profile fits you it is time for you to seek an understanding of why you are using food as a weapon against yourself. Remember, guns don't kill, just the person who pulls the trigger. Therefore, it is not the food that is at fault but rather the person who is putting it in his or her mouth. If you can honestly rationalise why you seek refuge in eating you will then have the opportunity to remove the cause and positively change your life. If the cause is not readily apparent to you it is highly probable you are harbouring a deep seated psychosis which may require professional help to uncover.

Adapting to a healthy lifestyle

Until such time as dietary change becomes a universal happening you may be seen as the odd person out, and this will be your greatest test. Most people who modify their diet to exclude junk food lose the desire to eat junk food, but guilt is their sworn enemy. Being unable to say no for fear of offending your host is something you will have to learn to deal with. But, as you are permitted access to a such a wide range of foods under the *Slim Forever* program, offending your host will be unlikely if you are tactful.

The Reverend Trevor Loveday of Sydney gave an account of how he coped with eating in restaurants and in other people's homes during his period of **Slim Forever** weight loss. Initially he was sensitive about offending his hosts, but he soon discovered it was his sensitivity and not that of his hosts that was at issue. If he was required to eat lunch in a restaurant he would order, for instance, fish without salad or vegetables which would satisfy both his hunger and the requirements of his weight loss program. He countered questions such as, 'Aren't you having anything else?' with a polite 'No thank you, this is what I eat for lunch', and the subject was immediately forgotten.

Mass education toward better nutrition is a difficult task, especially when more money is spent on advertising junk food than any other commodity. There is no money to be made from good nutrition and balanced eating, but there is a fortune to be plucked from selling junk food. When was the last time you saw an advertisement urging you to cook a steak and make a fresh garden salad with homemade dressing?

Nutritionally balanced food satisfies the hunger and is not addictive, unlike sugar-based foods which some people consume until they become ill. Poor nutrition and poor health are a bonanza for junk food and drug manufacturers who spend billions of dollars annually to keep us that way.

Who is responsible?

Being slim is a question of responsibility. Your health and your well-being are your concern and not the concern of any other person. There is not another soul who can take the initiative to transform you into a healthier and happier person. You alone must accept the responsibility for your present physical condition and only you can institute any meaningful change. Other people in your life will benefit from you becoming a slimmer and healthier person, but the person who will really benefit is you. If you have forgotten how it feels to be slim and totally alive, you are missing out on one of the greatest experiences life can offer.

Your **Slim Forever** program will be your passport to a slimmer, healthier and happier life. This is something you can do for yourself, so reach out and embrace it. You will be glad you did.

IS AGE A BARRIER TO LOSING WEIGHT?

No! Definitely not.

There are many misconceptions involving the human body and the ageing process. Suggesting older people quite naturally put on weight as a matter of course just happens to be one of them.

The ageing process is as much a state of mind as it is a state of biological reality. There are some people who have themselves convinced they are old at 40, yet there are those who believe they are still teenagers when they are in their eighties. Many people spend their entire lives avoiding exercise, and ageing becomes a convenient excuse. A positive attitude, a good diet, and regular exercise are the three magic components of healthy ageing.

The accumulation of excess body fat is directly proportional to a person's intake of fat forming foods, and to the level of energy output. As our appetites seldom decline along with a decline in our relative levels of physical activity, the human body, irrespective of its biological age, has no option other than to store the overabundance of food as unused energy in the form of fat.

The ageing process is a direct result of mutational changes to the 75 trillion cells comprising the structure of the human body. There are many agents external to the body which contribute significantly to these changes, including, but certainly not limited to, ultraviolet light, infection, pharmaceuticals and toxic chemicals. These toxic agents each in their own way contribute to the ageing process by adversely influencing the genetic coding contained within each functional cell.

From the first moments of embryonic conception, our bodies commence the lifelong process of cellular destruction and reconstruction which is the very basis of our existence. Each cell undergoing replacement initiates new cellular growth and reproduces itself in its own likeness, but if the host cell is damaged, those mutational faults will be implanted in the genetic coding of the newly forming cell. These many and often tiny mutations accumulate and eventually claim our lives, but the rate of accumulation is greatly influenced by the degree of abuse we level upon ourselves. You cannot reasonably expect to consistently abuse your body *and* live a long and healthy life.

Barring the unforeseen, the ageing cellular mutation process can be positively influenced by reducing the amount of toxic agents we ingest, by undertaking regular daily exercise and by eating a healthy and balanced diet.

With the exception of menarche and menopause in the female, the functions of the human body change little throughout the course of our lives. An older body will gain weight and get lazy just the same as a young body, but so too will it respond to positive change. The *Slim Forever* program is based on an appreciation of the quantity and balance of foods necessary to lose unwanted body fat, and keep it off, irrespective of age. If you are of mature age and overweight you can enjoy the benefits of being slimmer, healthier and happier by following this program, and by increasing your daily activity level.

Insomnia, constipation, osteoporosis and many of the aches and pains so often associated with ageing could largely be a thing of the past, but it is up to the individual to do something about it. Remember, you are only as old as you feel, and if you choose to sit around waiting to grow old, you certainly will, very quickly.

Your digestive system, your muscles and your overall energy level will respond positively to a balanced diet and a little daily exercise, regardless of your age. Life is for living, but you must put a little effort in if you expect to get something back, so give it a try. You have nothing to lose but your unwanted fat, your aches, your pains and your lack of energy!

5

why diets fail

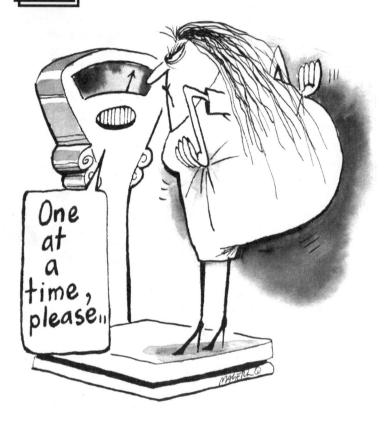

Is is water or is it fat?

Major causes of diet failure

Life after dieting

Potions, pills and promises

*If you subsist on alfalfa sprouts and wholegrain bread
you probably won't live longer, it will just seem like it.*

Jane Frazer, 1992

People in the United States are currently spending an estimated $18 billion annually in their bid to lose unwanted body fat. Figures are not available for many of the other industrialised countries, but the total worldwide expenditure on diet and slimming programs must be staggering. The need for an effective and sustainable weight loss program is well demonstrated, yet statistically, commercial diets are abysmal failures. As few as 3% of all people embarking on diets actually reach their desired level of weight loss *and* maintain it.

There is certainly no lack of players in the diet vending stakes. It is difficult to pick up a magazine, especially those aimed at the female reading market, without being confronted by yet another revolutionary diet. The sheer magnitude of the material must prompt the question – if just one of these diets worked, would there ever have been the need for another?

We have been assailed by a barrage of options including the grapefruit diet, the egg diet, the water diet, the banana diet, the rice diet and countless other diets based on the consumption of almost every single food or combination of foods known. There are diets based on the elimination of all meats in favour of fruit and vegetables, and diets that advocate the eating of meat to the exclusion of fruit and vegetables. The diets may differ, however, they all share the common denominator of starvation. If you reduce your intake of food sufficiently you will lose weight, of this there can be no argument. But, unless your diet optimises your daily allowable intake of carbohydrates, proteins and fats, the weight you lose may well represent body fluid and essential muscle tissue, and very little body fat.

IS IT WATER OR IS IT FAT?

The fact that your bathroom scale indicates a loss in overall body weight does not necessarily mean a reduction in body fat. Clinical studies involving weight loss due to starvation have produced some interesting results. In one such experiment six men starved for a period of 10 days, each losing an average of 16 lb/7.25 kg in body weight, but much of the weight lost was attributed to a loss of body fluids, not fat.

The greater part of your total body weight is water, estimated at between 50% and 60% in the healthy adult female, and between 60% and 70% in the healthy adult male. As water is a necessary component in the transport of glucose and triglycerides into the fat storage cells, fluid retention will increase with any increase in body fat deposits. Fluid increase under conditions of active fat formation can be as high as 40% in some individuals, and with many of us that means every day. Under extreme dietary conditions a considerable portion of this retained fluid will be expelled, a loss accounting for most of the recorded initial weight loss associated with many diets. Fluid loss due to starvation dieting will be quickly replaced when normal eating and drinking resumes. As most disillusioned dieters return to their previous eating habits, and very often with a vengeance, the fat formation and fluid retention process will be immediately restarted.

Once a body perceives starvation it will initiate steps to preserve stored fat by breaking down essential muscle tissue and converting it into glucose for energy. In the long-term, degraded skeletal muscle due to starvation seldom fully regenerates without the undertaking of resistance exercise. Repeated bouts of starvation dieting compound this problem. As muscle becomes the major source of energy, the reduction in muscle mass will result in a corresponding reduction in the future demand for glucose and fat for energy. The less energy fuel burned by the muscle, the greater will be the rate of conversion of excess glucose and dietary fats into body fat. This is the reason why periodic dieters progressively generate more body fat from the same quantity of food following each failed attempt at dieting.

The loss of muscle bulk associated with low protein dieting is not confined to muscle degradation for the production of energy. Any decrease in the consumption of protein below the optimum daily intake requirement will adversely affect the replacement of muscle as part of the normal life cycle. The absence of available protein to the regenerating muscle cells will abort the formation of body tissue, resulting in an overall loss of body weight. The author has recorded accelerated muscle regeneration of up to 6lb 8 oz/3 kg in just five days of consuming a balanced intake of protein following starvation dieting.

The problem of post-diet eating is all too often accompanied by a perceived sense of personal failure. Doubt and frustration associated with such failures frequently drive the disappointed dieter to overindulge in food in response to a subliminal desire for self-punishment to atone that failure.

MAJOR CAUSES OF DIET FAILURE

Statistically, 97% of all dieters fail in their quest to lose weight and to keep it off, and most will regain all of their lost weight, or more, within a two year period.

It is the balance rather than the quantity of the foods we eat that is responsible for the formation of excess body fat. The basis of most diets is an overall reduction in the amount of food consumed without alteration to the balance of those foods. By maintaining dietary imbalance the body is prevented from switching to burning fat for energy, and so the fat deposits are preserved. The often drastic reduction in food intake associated with many diets signals starvation and the body will move to preserve stored body fat at the expense of muscle. Also, a starving body will send conscious messages for food which are loud and clear, and difficult to ignore. So, unless you are prepared to keep yourself in a state of perpetual hunger, your attempts at dieting are guaranteed to fail.

The two major contributing factors to commercial diet failure are the lack of understanding of:

1 why a person accumulates excess body fat in the first place; and

2 what dietary changes are necessary to mobilise and reduce levels of stored body fat.

Carbohydrate is the major fat forming food of the human body, yet most diets recommend meals high in carbohydrate and low in protein. Although less efficient than fat, the body will choose carbohydrate (glucose) over stored fat for the production of energy if glucose is in abundance in the bloodstream. However, long-term excessive carbohydrate consumption does more than just overpower the body's fat burning potential. It actually creates a pathway for the burning of glucose which will eventually become dominant to the burning of fat, thereby altering the way the body produces energy. By merely reducing the overall intake of food, little else happens other than the body becomes starved of carbohydrate, protein and fat. And, as the metabolic pathway for energy production has been altered to burn predominantly glucose, the body will not turn to burning body fat, but will seek more glucose. This it acquires by switching immediately to the degradation of muscle and converting it into glucose. Once the breakdown of muscle commences, and this may only take three days of reduced food dieting, the body will move to preserve its stores of fat.

To be effective a weight loss program must first deliver a balance of foods capable of supplying the body with sufficient quantities of all of the essential nutrients. Secondly, it must be capable of retraining the body to again burn fat as its major energy source without signalling starvation. Then, and only then, will the body give up its deposits of fat, and preserve essential muscle.

LIFE AFTER DIETING

Another common problem with many weight loss programs is their failure to address the very important subject of weight maintenance once the primary period of dieting is completed. Simple logic dictates that if, after a period of dieting, a person returns to their original eating habits, then these same eating habits must again cause weight gain.

Weight maintenance can only be achieved if a balance of the three major food groups is sustained. But, as the loss of body fat is no longer actively sought during weight maintenance, the daily intake of carbohydrate can be increased by 50% under the *Slim Forever* program without again forming body fat.

POTIONS, PILLS AND PROMISES

No treatise on dieting would be complete without addressing the effects on the body of fat formation suppressors. There is little doubt a totally safe pill designed to keep us slim while we indiscriminately eat, drink and be merry would have widespread public appeal. Pills containing appetite suppressors such as caffeine have been around for years, but new breeds of pills are emerging.

Carbohydrate blockers

Pills known generically as carbohydrate blockers hit the market in the late 1980s. They came with a promise of freedom to eat all or anything a person wanted without the fat-forming carbohydrates ever being absorbed into the bloodstream. People flocked to buy them. The media reported lines of shoppers stretching for blocks outside some stores when these pills were released onto the North American market, but fortunately the United States Food and Drug Administration acted quickly to ban further sales.

Carbohydrate blockers were a potential health hazard of unimaginable proportions, and many deaths would have resulted had sales not been curtailed. A body totally starved of carbohydrate will revert to breaking down essential muscle tissue for the production of glucose. This in turn may lead to the possible production of ketone bodies in the bloodstream and the onset of a condition known as toxic ketosis. Ketone bodies are poisonous and will cause serious illness or even death if the concentration rises sufficiently.

Basal metabolic rate stimulants

Research is now focused on producing a pill designed to increase the amount of energy a body produces by artificially increasing the basal metabolic rate (BMR). The BMR is a function best described as the rate at which the physical and chemical processes of our body are maintained under conditions of load and stress.

At a conference on 'Obesity in the 21st Century' held in London in 1992, Professor Mike Stocks from London's St George's Hospital announced that the new generation drugs called *thermogenic b-3 agonists* could be on the market in a few years (*Sunday Telegraph,* 28 June 1992). These drugs are designed to artificially increase the BMR by stimulating the body's brown fat cells to produce additional body heat, thereby reducing body fat deposits. However, there is contention as to whether the adult human actually has brown fat cells. Some animals have large deposits of brown fat and are capable of increasing internal body heat (thermogenesis) by as much as 500% under conditions of extreme cold. But not so the adult human according to some authorities. Even under conditions of severe cold, the adult human can only stimulate thermogenesis by 10% to 15%, a sharp contrast to animals with a body heating system up to 50 times more efficient.

The human infant has a small amount of brown fat which is thought to be a necessary component in the maintenance of body temperature in the newborn. However, according to Dr Arthur C. Guyton, Professor and Chairman of the Department of Physiology and Biophysics at the University of Mississippi School of Medicine, the adult human has almost no brown fat. Even if sufficient brown fat was available for the stimulation of additional heat in the adult, what would be the total effect on the body?

The generic name assigned these new pills suggests they are being designed to stimulate (agonist) body heat (thermogenesis) by stimulating the recently discovered beta-3 (b-3) heat producing pathway. The production of body heat in response to a fall in external temperature is under the control of the hormones epinephrine, norepinephrine and thyroxine, which are coincidentally three in number. But, these hormones perform functions other than the production of heat. Epinephrine and norepinephrine also constrict blood vessels, increase heart activity, inhibit the function of the gastrointestinal tract, and dilate the pupils of the eyes. The hormone thyroxine stimulates protein and carbohydrate metabolism, calcium retention, bone growth, heart and respiration rates, muscle contraction and all communication between the brain and the body. It is also an important factor in the eradication of excess cholesterol, triglycerides, phospholipids and unwanted free fatty acids from the blood stream. Prolonged increases in thyroxine levels may give rise to constipation, increased arterial pressure, extreme nervousness, anxiety, paranoia and muscle tremors. If the proposed thermogenic b-3 agonists are designed to stimulate the production of any of these hormones to increase heat production, all other associated functions must also be affected.

Let us assume for a moment the chemical stimulation of the BMR of a person taking these new drugs was successful. What will become of the unwanted heat produced during that reaction? Our bodies react to overheating by transferring much of the excess heat to the skin surface where it is dissipated into the atmosphere. This is achieved by enlarging the pores of the skin and evaporating the surface moisture, or perspiration. Does it then follow that a person taking these drugs will constantly perspire?

The effects of prolonged chemically induced increases in body heat (hyperthermia) may create manifestly greater problems than those associated with being overweight or obese. Studies conducted in the United Kingdom in 1988 indicated an accelerated fat loss with some people taking thermogenic b-3 agonists in conjunction with a diet program. However, two-thirds of the test subjects presented with side effects, including hand tremors, causing the drug company owning the rights to the drug to abandon further development. Not surprisingly, testing is continuing with other companies lured by the enormous potential profits a marketable fat loss drug could bring.

Our bodies have been four million years in the making, and that is an awfully long time to survive without the availability of drugs in order to lose weight. You may effectively achieve your goal of losing unwanted body fat, and keeping it off, simply by balancing your intake of food as outlined in the *Slim Forever* program. What could be more natural?

6

don't count calories

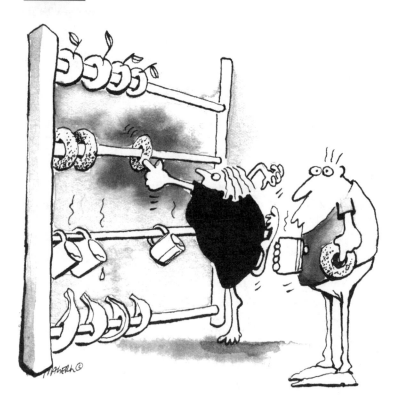

The doubtful measure

THE DOUBTFUL MEASURE

Calories represent a rather complex, but totally meaningless method of establishing the fat forming content of food. A calorie is the designated measure of a unit of heat, described as the quantity of heat required to raise the temperature of 1 g of pure water 1°C from a standard temperature (usually 3.98°C, 14.5°C, or 19.5°C) at sea level.

Not satisfied with calories, we have also adopted the International System unit of energy called a joule (J) which is described as being equal to the energy consumed when a current of 1 ampere of electricity is passed through a resistance equal to 1 ohm for a period of 1 second. The heat produced by 1 J is quite small, so, in an effort to make them more manageable, we group joules in lots of 1,000 and refer to them as kilojoules (kJ). If you wish to equate calories to joules, the heat produced by 1 calorie is equal to the heat produced by 4.184 J.

In an effort to rationalise the formation of unwanted body fat, researchers have attempted to establish just how much energy a particular food source contains, and just how much energy we expend undertaking certain activities. It was postulated that by understanding the exact relationship between the two, a diet linked to a person's particular activity level should eliminate the formation of excess body fat.

Energy is expressed as units of heat, therefore it was reasoned that:

1   by measuring the heat potential of every food; and

2   by measuring the heat produced by the body when converting those foods into energy,

it would be possible to establish a link between food intake and body energy production.

To determine the energy potential of a particular food, a specific portion of that food is burned in a calorimeter. The heat generated by the burning food becomes the calorific value of that particular food. The next step was to determine how much energy the human body uses when performing certain physical activities. This was achieved by measuring the heat of a body at rest, and again when the body was placed under load. The difference between the two recorded values represented the additional energy required to undertake that activity.

The object of the exercise was commendable, but, at no time has any apparent consideration been given to what happens to food from the various food groups once it enters the body.

The fate of dietary proteins

Protein is measured for its calorific value, but protein is used almost entirely in the reconstruction of almost every tissue in the human body other than bone. Seldom is protein used by the body for the production of energy. However, protein burned in a calorimeter does produce heat. This being the case, the calorific value of the protein we eat should be excluded from the evaluation process, but it isn't.

The fate of dietary carbohydrates

Carbohydrates supply the body with nothing other than energy producing sugars, but it is not just the sugar portion of the foods that undergo calorific heat analysis. Some carbohydrate foods contain little or no sugar, but they do contain a lot of indigestible fibre which burns and produces heat in the calorimeter. Of the foods we eat, especially high fibre carbohydrate foods, only a very small portion passes from the intestinal tract into the bloodstream. The bulk of all ingested solid food is expelled from the body as faecal material. Once again, a meaningful assessment of the energy potential of the foods we consume could only be made if the calorific value of the waste products from the body are first established, and this value deducted from the overall equation.

The fate of dietary fats

Fats too are included in the evaluation process, but fats and oils, be they saturated or unsaturated, have functions other than the production of body energy. Unsaturated fats contain linoleic, linolenic and arachidonic acids, essential ingredients in the structural development of cell membranes, in the promotion of blood clotting and in the manufacture of prostaglandins. Fats are involved in the production of nerve tissue, skin, some hormones and in the formation of a protective shock-absorbing layer around some organs. They are important factors in the development of sexual maturation, in pregnancy, in the formation of maternal milk and in the synthesis of bile salts, lipoproteins and cholesterol. Not one of these important functions involves any appreciable production of heat. Any fats so used must therefore be discounted from the equation if a true appreciation of their involvement in the production of body energy is to be established.

At no time has any attempt been made to establish the non-energy producing roles of proteins, carbohydrates or fats. Consequently, dietary recommendations are made based on the calorific content of foods which have no bearing whatsoever on the potential of those foods to produce energy, or body fat.

Other questions must also be answered.

Q *Does the fat formed from the excessive consumption of glucose, proteins or fats have the same potential to produce body energy as its component parts in the calorimeter?*

For example, stored fat has an energy potential $2\frac{1}{4}$ times greater than the energy potential of glucose. Therefore, the energy produced from glucose immediately entering the body would be manifestly less than energy produced from the same glucose once it had undergone transformation into body fat. The task of distinguishing between the percentage of ingested carbohydrate used immediately for energy production, and the percentage converted into fat for energy, would be an impossible one.

Q *Although derived from the same source, does the fat used for warming the body generate more radiant heat than the fat used in the production of muscle contractile energy?*

On a cold day a body at rest will commence shivering in an effort to produce body heat, an action quite different from the contraction of muscles under physical load. The action of shivering involves short rapid contractions of muscles not under load, with minimal energy being diverted into contractile energy and a maximum of energy being converted into body heat. Conversely, a muscle under physical load will convert the majority of the available energy into contractile energy, with only a small amount being expended on the production of heat. Energy can only be used once, and the available energy for the contraction of muscles, or shivering, is no exception. It would then follow that the external recording of body temperature would not be able to differentiate between the amount of energy involved in producing body heat, and the amount of energy involved in contracting muscles.

Q *How does the calorific evaluation distinguish between the various types of food?*

Perhaps the greatest failing of calorific food evaluation is the system's inability to differentiate between the various food sources. A diet may suggest the consumption of a maximum of 1500 calories each day without suggesting a balance in the foods consumed. For instance, if you consumed your allotted quota of 1500 calories in the form of sugar, your body would be starved of essential proteins, fats, and many essential vitamins and minerals. And further, if the ingested sugar exceeds the body's immediate carbohydrate requirement, the excess would be converted into stored fat. Alternatively, if you consumed just proteins and/or fats to the exclusion of carbohydrates, your body would initiate the conversion of muscle into glucose. As the energy produced from glucose due to the degradation of muscle did not form part of the original 1500 calorie assessment, the association between the food consumed and the generation of body energy cannot be validated.

Q *What has the measurement of heat, based on the determination of energy involved in raising the temperature of water, or by passing electricity through a barrier, got to do with the fat forming content of the foods we eat?*

The answer is, absolutely nothing.

Your **Slim Forever** program offers perhaps the only safe and scientifically based assessment of the foods you eat. The balance between proteins, carbohydrates and fats takes into account nutritional content, absorption ratios, and body utilisation under all conditions of physical activity.

For the sake of your health, **don't count calories!**

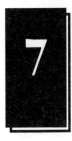

7

digestion and the hunger response

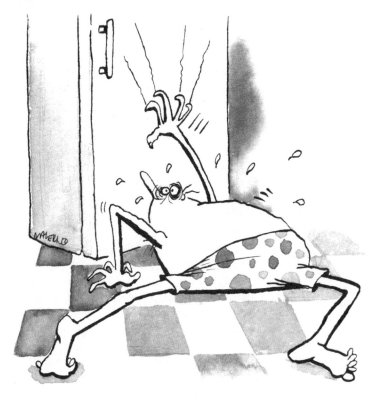

An insight into digestion

The hunger response

AN INSIGHT INTO DIGESTION

Digestion is the process employed by our bodies which prepares the food we eat in readiness for the extraction of nutrients essential to human growth and survival.

The food we eat passes through the digestive tract, which is little more than a sophisticated tube extending from the input end, the mouth, to the output end, the anus. The digestive tract is comprised of three major portions, the stomach, the small intestine and the large intestine or colon, with each portion performing a specialised function. Technically, the inside of the digestive tract forms part of the outside of the body, a little like the hole in a doughnut. Because of its length, approximately 26 ft/8 m in the average adult, it is wound around in the abdomen rather like a randomly coiled rope. As food travels along this tube the nutrients contained within that food are absorbed through the wall of the intestine and into the body proper. The bulk of the food itself is not absorbed, just the essential nutrients it contains, and the residue is passed out of the body as faecal material.

How is food digested?

The digestive process starts in the mouth where the food we eat is physically reduced in size to more manageable pieces by the process of chewing, or mastication. The presence of food in the mouth initiates the production of saliva, and the first of the digestive enzymes, ptyalin. The act of swallowing causes the now masticated food to drop down into the sack-like stomach, the major area of pre-digestion. Special cells in the wall of the stomach produce highly concentrated hydrochloric acid and other enzymes, which are the necessary agents for the pre-digestion of proteins, carbohydrates and fats. The remainder of the cells in the stomach are bathed in a special fluid which makes them resistant to the eroding effects of the digestive fluids.

Water plays a significant role in the absorption of nutrients, but as the fats we eat are not soluble in water, they require special treatment. Water solubility of dietary fat is achieved by adding emulsifying agents in the form of bile salts. Bile salts are produced by the liver and stored in the gall bladder and are released on demand via the common bile duct into the stomach.

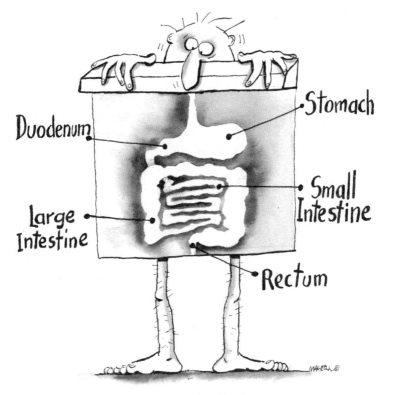

The Digestive System
Figure 19.2

The pre-digested food, now referred to as food bolus, starts its journey into the small intestine. But first, it passes through a smaller pouch, the duodenum, where an alkaline solution is added to neutralise the potential burning effects of any residual hydrochloric acid.

The food bolus now enters the small intestine where the absorption of nutrients begins, along with the absorption of many other not so desirable food additives and toxic substances. The intestine's potential to absorb nutrients is directly proportional to its surface area, which in a smooth tube would be minimal. To increase its absorption capabilities the inside wall of the small intestine is covered with millions of tightly packed finger-like projections called villi which protrude out into the mass of food bolus.

The wall of the intestine is largely constructed of muscle, and the food bolus is moved along the intestine by a rippling contraction of the muscles of the intestine, called peristalsis. This action is very controlled and unidirectional, similar to that of a caterpillar crawling. In addition to propelling the food along the length of the intestine, this rippling action also churns the food over and over like concrete in a mixer. This ensures most of the food bolus makes contact with the nutrient absorption surface of the intestine. As only those nutrients coming into physical contact with the wall of the intestine can be absorbed, the action of peristalsis becomes extremely important in the digestive process.

The molecules of pre-digested minerals, chemicals, proteins, sugars and fats are absorbed through pores in the intestinal villi and into the bloodstream. The bloodstream is really the urban transit system of the body, carrying nutrients and oxygen to the cells and returning with the metabolic waste products. It collects its load of nutrients from the inner surface of the small intestine, oxygen from the lungs and hormones from other organs. The metabolic waste products are deposited in the kidneys for eradication in the urine.

The absorption of fluids

Fluids are also absorbed through the intestinal wall and deposited into the bloodstream. Therefore, almost all of whatever you drink must enter the bloodstream before it can again be expelled from the body. The body regulates the amount of fluid it retains by passing the blood through the kidneys where the excess fluid is extracted and passed out as urine. Ingested fluid is essential for the replacement of body fluid lost through natural evaporation and dehydration, and also as a vehicle for the expulsion of waste products from the inner body. The kidneys are the clearing houses of most blood borne toxins and of cellular waste, the by-products of normal metabolic activity. With too little disposable fluid in the blood, these waste products become concentrated, and may actually poison the body.

However, too great an intake of fluids can also be harmful. The fluids we drink dilute the blood, and if taken to excess can reduce the concentration of the oxygen and essential nutrients it carries. Diluted concentrations of nutrients and oxygen demand an increase in the rate at which the blood flows, and this the body achieves by increasing the heart rate. A prolonged increase in heart rate due to sustained excessive fluid in the blood translates into greater pressure being exerted on the heart and the arteries, a condition known as hypertension. Hypertension can result from a number of pathological conditions, including of course, heart failure and kidney dysfunction. Those of us who drink fluids to excess, be it water, milk, juice, soft drink, tea, coffee or alcohol usually maintain at least a moderate level of self-induced hypertension, which will in time take its toll. Therefore, the sensible control of fluid intake is as important in the regulation of good health as is the sensible control of solid food consumption.

The body's waste management system

At the distal end of the 20 ft/6 m long small intestine, the now nutrient depleted food bolus moves into the large intestine or colon. Apart from some salt, fluid and vitamins B and K absorption, the large intestine plays no role in nutrient uptake. The function of the colon is the transformation by bacterial action of the spent food bolus into faecal material in preparation for its expulsion from the body. It is not fully understood why the body goes to such lengths in this degradation process, but so intense is the bacterial action that fully one-third of the bulk of faecal discharge is active bacteria, or flora.

Why no safety valve?

The human nutrient absorption system is relatively simple in both design and operation, but we do lack one very important function. Unfortunately we are not fitted with a limiting device capable of restricting nutrient absorption once the body has taken its fill, and probably for very good reason. In ages past when regular meals did not form part of the daily routine, the body would store any excess of nutrients during feasting, and use them during times of famine.

Although our eating habits have changed, the basic functions of our bodies have not. The more we eat, the more nutrients our bodies will absorb, and if these nutrients are not fully expended, the more stored fat we will accumulate. We could of course revert to form, and engorge ourselves on a leg of beef for a day or two, and totally starve for the next four or five. However, it is highly unlikely any of us would choose that option. Alternatively, we could balance our intake of food to coincide with our own particular energy production and body building requirements, and avoid forming excess fat in the first place.

Your body has no option other than to process every single morsel of food you put in your mouth, be it nutritional, or just plain junk. Be sensible about what you eat and drink, and look after your body. It is the only one you will ever have.

THE HUNGER RESPONSE

The hunger response is our body's way of telling us we are in need of nutritional sustenance. Just as the pain response signals something is amiss with our body, and abdominal discomfort alerts us of the need to evacuate waste, our body signals the need for food. But, in all cases these responses can be manipulated.

The body has two opposing responses relative to eating. The first is the hunger response which alerts us of the conscious need to consume food. The second is the satiety response which tells us to stop eating. Both of these responses are initiated individually by the brain from a specific area called the hypothalamus.

Quantity response

When the body requires food, it signals a conscious desire to eat by stimulating the hunger response, suppressing the satiety response and initiating rhythmic contractions of the stomach. If ignored, for whatever reason, these contractions can become so intense as to cause mild pain, a condition we generally refer to as hunger pangs. A hungry person deprived of food may also experience the onset of tension and restlessness, and a feeling of strangeness and nausea throughout the entire body, symptoms that will only be satisfied by eating.

Quality response

In addition to the hunger or quantity response, we also have an appetite or quality response. This expresses itself as a desire for specific types of food. It is designed to alert us to the need for certain nutrients the body considers essential at that precise time. If you have tried dieting on just fruit and salads, and experienced the burning desire for a steak, you will have experienced the quality response. It was not just your feeling of deprivation for real food that triggered the craving, but more probably the body telling you it needed protein.

Programming the quality response

The appetite response is influenced by the impact on the body of the foods we eat and the liquids we drink. Our reaction to each dietary experience is recorded by the brain in a similar manner to the storing of data in a computer. This accumulative programming response commences the moment we are born. Sigmund Freud referred to the period of infant development when everything goes into the mouth as the oral stage, a time when taste is the dominant vehicle of learning.

Any exposure of the senses to the sight, sound, smell, touch or taste of any food will trigger a data search in the brain. If located, the relevant information will immediately be brought forward into the conscious mind. Each specific programmed memory response is predicated on the perceived positive or negative nature of each prior experience. An experience may be classified as being good or bad, or it may only provoke a response of indifference. Young children often fail to register any apparent repulsion, even to the most repugnant of sampled items. This apparent absence of reaction has nothing to do with poor taste evaluation, but everything to do with a lack of prior eating and taste experience. In time, the child's brain will register pleasure or repugnance, and a corresponding positive or negative response to repeated taste exposure will be initiated.

There is no apparent reason why individuals react differently to the same food source. Oysters are a prime example. People either love them or hate them, there is usually no middle ground. We may, as individuals, share many similar taste traits with others, but few people are identical in their appreciation of food. The forcing of an individual, especially a child, to eat a particular food just because it is considered healthy or palate pleasing by the protagonist, may do more harm than good to the development of taste appreciation in that child. The forced eating of food deemed by the recipient to be distasteful tends to reinforce the programmed rejection, not reduce it.

As we advance into adulthood we continue to program new food reaction responses. Exposure to a food we have not previously encountered will elicit a blank response from the brain. Unless we perceive the food as looking or smelling bad, we will need to taste it in order to gain a programmable response. The new programming response commences immediately the food enters the mouth. Rejection by expectoration may be immediate if the taste or texture of the food are not immediately appealing. If not, the food will be accepted and swallowed, and the stomach will have the option of retaining or rejecting it. If either the taste or swallowing experience is perceived as being bad, your brain will raise a red flag next time you are confronted with that particular food. Conversely, if the new food passes all of the required sight, smell and taste tests, the response recorded will be positive and there will be a desire to consume that particular food again.

System failure

Unfortunately we can override any one or all of the hunger, satiety and appetite responses. This will in turn affect our judgment as to the quality and the quantity of the food we eat. Constant and indiscriminate eating will eventually rob us of the ability to experience real hunger, or to know when we have had enough to eat. But, more importantly, any person who constantly overeats usually loses the ability to differentiate between good and bad foods.

Sugar is the trigger

As is the case with most brain responses, stimulus from another part of the body is usually necessary to initiate activity. In the case of hunger and satiety, the initiating factor for both responses is the perceived level of glucose in the blood. Decreased blood glucose will signal a need for nutritional sustenance by increasing the magnitude of the electrical responses to the hunger centre while decreasing the magnitude of the electrical responses to the satiety centre. These concurrent signals simultaneously increase hunger and decrease satiety, resulting in a perceived need to eat.

Immediately ingested sugar enters the bloodstream, blood glucose levels will rise and a reverse of the above actions will occur. An adequate blood glucose level will initiate a decrease in the hunger response and a corresponding increase in the satiety response, signalling a need to stop eating.

Design and function of the human body are absolutes, and so too are the hunger and satiety co-responses — responses that work exceptionally well, provided we don't change the rules. The protracted change in diet to include more carbohydrate has struck at the very core of the hunger response, creating a condition known as the hyper-hypoglycaemic swing, a condition responsible for exciting hunger and reducing satiety out of all proportion.

Appetites out of control

It is reasonable to assume that the more carbohydrate we eat, the greater will be the suppressive action on the hunger response, and the greater will be the corresponding excitation of the satiety response. But, this is not the case. The end product of all the carbohydrate we consume is glucose, a necessary form of fuel for the production of energy in the human body. However, there are definite limits as to how much glucose a body can store and use before any excess to immediate requirements is converted into stored fat.

Glucose in the bloodstream is a potential fuel source. It only becomes actively involved in producing energy once it gains entry into the muscle and tissue cells. This it achieves with the assistance of insulin, a hormone produced by the pancreas in amounts proportional to the concentration of glucose in the blood. Under balanced eating conditions, any rise or fall in the production of insulin could be best described as a gentle ebb and flow. However, if the levels of glucose in the blood suddenly become excessively high, in a condition known as hyperglycaemia, insulin production will undergo rapid acceleration. Once initiated, the accelerated production of insulin will persist at the elevated level for as long as excessive blood glucose is detected.

Unfortunately, the production of insulin does not cease as soon as the level of blood glucose returns to normal. Due to a lag in time between the pancreas perceiving a reduction in blood glucose and its ability to initiate a slowing of insulin production, there is an abnormally high production of surplus insulin produced. As insulin has an irreversible attraction to glucose, the surplus insulin continues to attach itself to whatever glucose it can find, removing it from the bloodstream. This results in an overabsorption of glucose from the bloodstream, and the onset of low blood sugar, or hypoglycaemia.

What does all this mean? Simply put, the consumption of carbohydrates, especially foods containing refined sugar, will throw the body's normal hunger and satiety responses out of kilter. Instead of feeling satisfied with what you have eaten, low blood glucose levels caused by an overproduction of insulin will soon have you craving for food your body does not need.

Nature's appetite suppressors

Insulin plays only a minor role in the metabolic uptake of both protein and fat by the cells. As the consumption of meat and dairy products does not initiate insulin production, the hunger response will be suppressed.

It is ironical, but sad, that most diets stress the need for an increase in carbohydrate foods such as fruit, vegetables and grain products, all of which:

1 stimulate the hunger response;

2 suppress the mobilisation of stored body fat; and

3 contribute more to the formation of fat on the human body than any other food source.

Sugar diabetes

The overproduction of insulin due to excessive sugar intake places an unreasonable load on the beta cells of the pancreas. In time, a forced production schedule may lead to a decline in the production of insulin and to the onset of insulin deficient diabetes. If your diet is dominated by carbohydrate foods and you become light-headed and crave something sweet every couple of hours, you are on a collision course with your pancreas.

Six out of every ten people in the industrialised world are borderline or active diabetics, simply because they have for too long been consuming too much sugar.

Conversely, protein and fat actively suppress the hunger response and excite the satiety response, thereby effectively reducing the perceived need to eat. If not consumed to excess, all protein will be totally consumed in tissue reconstruction, and all fat in the production of energy and the mobilisation of stored body fat. As protein and fat make no demand on the pancreas for the production of insulin, the problem of sugar induced diabetes could reasonably be eradicated.

The currently accepted protocol in treating hyperglycaemia involves a reduction in the consumption of proteins, with an emphasis on the consumption of carbohydrates. Eating is encouraged every few hours, and oral or intramuscular insulin is administered in advanced cases. Unfortunately this protocol is adding to, and not subtracting from the problem by stimulating the need for insulin from cells which are no longer capable of full production. A number of diagnosed diabetics suffering from dietary induced diabetes mellitus have adopted the *Slim Forever* program under the strict supervision of the author, and in every case the individual's blood sugar levels has been stabilised within a matter of days.

However, medication dependant diabetics should heed the warning in the front of this book before undertaking any dietary change.

Diabetes mellitus

This is a condition usually associated with impaired insulin production due to chronic excessive sugar ingestion. This is by far the most common form of diabetes and it will usually respond positively to controlled decreases in carbohydrate. However, any decrease in carbohydrate must be accompanied by a corresponding and supervised reduction in oral or intramuscular insulin. The administration of too much insulin may give rise to insulin acidosis, or insulin shock.

Conversely, the over-consumption of carbohydrate and too little insulin may give rise to excessively high levels of blood sugar and the onset of diabetic coma. Again, this condition will respond well to the controlled intake of carbohydrate.

Diabetes insipidus

Although a member of the diabetes family, diabetes insipidus does not involve insulin. It is a pathological condition in which there is a decrease in the production of antidiuretic hormone and an increase in urination. As insulin and sugar are not influencing factors, alterations in carbohydrate intake may be undertaken.

Hyperinsulinism

A much rarer condition, hyperinsulinism is usually associated with malignant or benign tumours of the pancreas. Insulin production dramatically increases and requires the constant administration of glucose to prevent insulin shock.

This condition *will not* respond favourably to decreases in carbohydrate consumption.

8

eating disorders

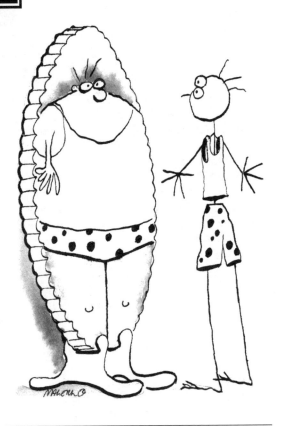

Fasting and starvation

Anorexia nervosa

Bulimia

FASTING AND STARVATION

In the practical sense, fasting and starvation are synonymous terms. Fasting is the act of voluntarily abstaining from eating, a decision often motivated by religious or perceived health obligations. Starvation is usually associated with the deprivation of food due to the existence of uncontrollable external influences imposed by nature, or at the hands of another. Irrespective of the influence, the effect on the body remains the same.

Positive scientific data relative to fasting is unavailable, however, the condemnation of fasting by most nutritionists is widespread. In addressing obesity, the Professor of Nutrition at Harvard University School of Public Health, Dr Jean Mayer writes: "I have been unimpressed with total fasting as a therapeutic measure. Published reports, including reports of accidents during total fasting, do not impel me to look at this method favourably." This opinion is supported by Dr Sue Rodwell Williams of the Kaiser-Permanente Medical Center in Oakland, California, who addresses the treatment of obesity during rehabilitation. She writes: "Indiscriminate fasting programs are unwise" and "a large part of the loss in such programs is only temporary water loss".

Claims made by proponents of fasting that abstinence from eating will result in loss of body fat or in a reduction of body toxicity are made totally without credible supportive evidence. Firstly, a starving body will quickly switch from burning fat to almost exclusively burning glucose and muscle for energy, thereby preserving the existing levels of body fat, not reducing them. Secondly, as most toxic chemicals find their way into the fat storage cells of our bodies, the eradication of these substances is hampered by fasting induced immobilisation of body fat. Detoxification is best achieved by removing further exposure to toxic contamination, and by balancing the diet so as to achieve optimum body function and fat mobilisation.

For some considerable time, the scientific community has relied on the results of tests involving laboratory rats to establish the effects of starvation. Unfortunately this is no longer the case as the world in recent years has been exposed to the reality of human starvation in a number of countries. The full spectrum of the effects of total starvation on humans is now, tragically, well understood.

Our bodies have three major nutrient group requirements, namely protein, fat and carbohydrate, along with a necessary complement of vitamins and minerals. A deficiency in any one nutrient group will result in some level of total body starvation, but a prolonged deficiency of all three will inevitably spell disaster.

The effects of starvation

The moment a body perceives the onset of starvation it immediately initiates steps to preserve essential body function. The widely held belief that carbohydrate is the major energy source is a hypothesis not shared by the body itself. Fat is the major energy source, and immediately the body senses starvation, it will move to preserve its precious stores of body fat, irrespective of the amounts held in storage. That is to say, an athlete with a ratio of 4% body fat to total body weight and an obese individual with a 50% body fat ratio would simultaneously enter the fat preservation mode under similar circumstances of starvation.

Once the preservation of stored body fat is initiated, the body will immediately turn to burning everything else at its disposal for energy, including all immediate stores of quickly expendable glucose and glycogen, and finally, muscle. The first outwardly apparent sign of starvation is muscle wasting due to the effect of a process referred to as gluconeogenesis. This involves the conversion of free protein and healthy muscle into glucose which is then burned in the energy production cycle.

Without food, the loss of essential muscle will continue unchecked due to the absence of muscle building protein and energy producing carbohydrate and fat. Starvation induced lethargy, a by-product of muscle wasting, will in turn develop into total body immobility. This is due in part to advanced skeletal muscle wasting, as well as an overall reduction in the availability of energy fuel. Even in a healthy body, glucose lacks the robust power of fat as an energy source, providing energy principally at the low exertion end of the physical activity scale. As gluconeogenesis produces only limited amounts of glucose, and in the almost total absence of available fat for energy, the starving body is forced to rely on extremely limited supplies of low energy glucose.

With time, the starving body will suffer the effects of vitamin and mineral deficiency. The body loses the ability to synthesise many hormones and essential enzymes, and this in turn will lead to widespread systems' malfunction. Poisons and waste products are no longer expelled from the body and the blood becomes highly toxic. In the advanced stages of starvation the body will lapse into a coma followed by total body shutdown. From this moment on the body will never again accept or process food, be it administered orally or intravenously.

Many commercial diets subscribe to the starvation principle. Although the effects are seldom fatal in the short-term, long-term muscle wasting and organ damage can, and usually does, occur following prolonged or repeated bouts with such diets.

ANOREXIA NERVOSA

The term anorexia simply means loss of appetite, but anorexia nervosa signifies a loss of appetite due to a serious mental disorder.

Anorexia nervosa is directly related to a person's mental perception of themselves as being overweight. The sufferer may not necessarily be overweight to any great degree, but develops a psychological fixation that he or she is overweight to such an extent that normal dieting soon gives way to self-imposed starvation. While not necessarily seeking to starve, anorexics become hapless victims to their insatiable quest for slimness.

Although anorexia nervosa affects some males, it has largely become a disease of young females. Reported cases in industrialised countries are increasing, with an estimated 15% of the young female population being affected to some degree. Tragically, this condition is needlessly claiming girls as young as eight years of age.

Much of the blame for this sudden upsurge of self-destructive dieting can be laid directly at the feet of the media and its many advertisers who seek to perpetuate the illusion that to be ultra slim is to be beautiful. In a recent study conducted in Britain a group of men and women were asked to self-evaluate their physical appearance and self-esteem. Following exposure to media photographs of models of similar age, all participants downgraded their perception of both their physical appearance and their self-esteem. However, exploitation of the ultra slim image appears to have gone full circle. Some actors, including the very people chosen to create the ultra-slim illusion, are falling victim to anorexia nervosa in a vain effort to retain viewers' acceptability and their jobs.

There is a fine psychological line separating the anorexia nervosa sufferer from the objective dieter. Objective dieters usually speak openly of their endeavour, whereas the anorexic will engage in devious deception to hide his or her affliction. The noticeable signs of this illness include:

1 making excuses to miss meals;

2 toying with food on the plate while eating very little; and

3 the undertaking of excessive exercise.

The anorexic will develop a washed-out complexion, and the skin will take on an almost transparent texture. Overt signs of advanced emaciation may soon follow.

Anorexia nervosa is a serious eating disorder with deep psychological overtones which if left unchecked may result in total starvation.

BULIMIA

The term bulimia specifically refers to any abnormal increase in the sensation of hunger, but it is now widely accepted as meaning forced overeating. Bulimia is a condition involving the constant and uncontrolled eating of food followed by induced vomiting or defecation, or both. Unlike the anorexic who takes little or no food, the bulimic engorges him or herself, and then purges the food from the body before it can be digested.

A form of bulimia was practised by the Court of the early Roman Empire where food, wine and sexual excesses were considered the right of the privileged class. Banquet halls were built with holes in the marble floor, appropriately placed beside each diner, into which the honoured guests would regurgitate undigested food, and recommence eating.

The true bulimic becomes emaciated in a similar fashion to the anorexic, but as some food invariably enters the digestive tract, protracted starvation may not be as readily apparent. The condition of bulimia typically goes undetected by others until it reaches an advanced stage.

Generally, a bulimic will display greater personal despair than the anorexic. Anorexia sufferers seek ultimate slimness, and a continuation of life, whereas the bulimic will often consider life to be devoid of any meaningful future. Eating to the bulimic is the weapon of choice in seeking release from an overwhelming obsession with poor self-esteem. The possibility of an early death is a reality, and perhaps may even be considered desirable by many victims.

Long-term anorexia nervosa and bulimia each rob the body of essential life-giving nutrients. Chronic calcium deprivation gives rise to bone and muscle weakness, and a lack of dietary phosphates often promotes kidney and heart failure. Both diseases are equally life-threatening, and should be viewed accordingly. If treatment is to be successful, professional psychological help, and the uncompromising support and understanding of family and friends are essential.

9

proteins, carbohydrates and fats

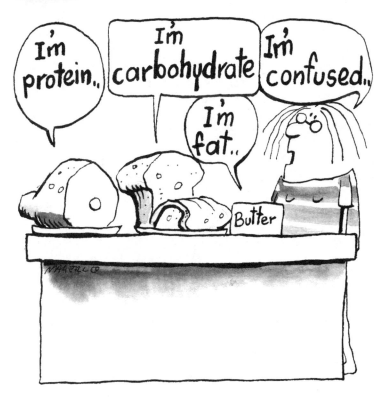

Proteins, carbohydrates and fats constitute the three major food sources of the human body. Although each group functions specifically, no one group is more important than another, with each playing a role in the absorption and utilisation process of its counterparts. To eliminate, reduce or excessively increase consumption of any one or any combination of the members of this group is to oppose the natural development and function of the human body, and to invite dietary disaster.

The motivating force behind most deviations from a naturally balanced diet do not necessarily come from a rational understanding of how the human body functions. We are by design omnivores, which simply means we eat food from both the meat and the vegetable groups. The digestive systems of omnivores are unique, as are the digestive systems of the meat eating carnivores and the vegetable eating herbivores. We cannot be compared to meat eating animals such as lions and tigers because of our dietary need for carbohydrate. Nor can we be compared to herbivores like cattle or elephants, due to our dietary need for meat and fat. A cow will not eat meat, a lion will not eat grass, and we must eat both, simply because each species has undergone specialised development under very different circumstances.

PROTEINS

Proteins exist in every known life form, both animal and vegetable. They represent the structural component of the human body, accounting for 75% of our dry soft tissue weight.

The number of individual proteins existing on this planet defies comprehension. Despite the enormity of their numbers, proteins are chains of small building blocks called amino acids of which there are just 19.

Amino acids

Each protein chain is identifiable by its specific number, combination and sequence of the amino acids forming its structure, a coding sequence not shared by other protein chains. The number of amino acids involved in the structure of a protein can range from just a few, to thousands, but not all proteins contain all 19 amino acids.

Complete and incomplete proteins

If a protein chain does contain all 19 amino acids it is classified as being a complete protein. Proteins with less than a full complement of amino acids are appropriately classified as being incomplete proteins. Complete proteins have the ability to supply the body with all of the building blocks necessary for total tissue growth and reconstruction. Theoretically, incomplete proteins can support body growth and reconstruction. However, for this to be a reality, a variety of incomplete proteins, each containing amino acids missing from their counterparts, must be consumed simultaneously and in sufficient quantities. Practically, this is not the case. Although many vegetables contain protein, it is typically low in concentration and usually incomplete. We simply do not have the human capacity to consume a cross-section of selected vegetables in sufficient quantities to satisfy our daily dietary protein needs.

Essential and non-essential amino acids

In addition to the classification of protein chains as being complete or incomplete, the amino acids themselves are classified as being either essential, or non-essential. Eight of the 19 amino acids cannot be produced internally by the human body, and it is therefore essential they be supplied from dietary sources. The remaining 11 amino acids can be synthesised by the human body, but only from other amino acids. These are classified as being non-essential. However, the ability of the body to synthesise non-essential amino acids is not a principal function. This is a backup system designed to satisfy the body's immediate need for amino acids during times of inadequate dietary protein intake. Ideally, all 19 amino acids should be consumed in the diet on a daily basis.

The digestion of proteins

By the addition of enzymes and acids in the mouth and stomach during digestion, the proteins we eat are almost entirely reduced from their complex chains to individual amino acids. Once absorbed into the bloodstream they join the metabolic pool of amino acids within the cells, there to await selection in the body building process.

Our bodies are in a constant state of destruction (catabolism) and reconstruction (anabolism) with all of the estimated 75 trillion cells undergoing constant replacement according to a specific order. When a cell dies, some of the still functional amino acids forming its structure are released back into the metabolic pool, and the non-reuseable amino acids are destroyed. The shortfall in amino acids created by this process, especially those classified as essential amino acids, must be replaced from ingested dietary protein.

To be effective, all 19 amino acids must be present in the metabolic pool at the precise moment a cell undertakes reconstruction. If a cell is seeking to manufacture a protein chain and just one of the amino acids is absent from the metabolic pool, the cell will abort the entire process. The body will then have to do without that particular protein until such time as the metabolic pool is replenished with the missing amino acid. This is known as the all or none principle.

Protein storage

Protein cannot be stored within the human body in any appreciable quantity. It must be consumed at regular intervals in amounts proportional to the individual's body size and physical work load. So critical is the need for a constant supply of protein, tissue rebuilding will be adversely affected within just four to six hours of consuming a meal deficient in one or more of those amino acids. Conversely, any protein consumed in excess of daily requirement may be converted into energy by the tissue cells.

A further complication is the formation of body fat from an abundance of some amino acids, even though a person may be generally protein deficient. If a particular amino acid is in abundance, but protein synthesis is aborted due to the absence of other amino acids, the amino acid in abundance will likely be converted into fat. Therefore, those who rely on incomplete protein from vegetables and grains may well be forming very little essential body protein, and a lot of unwanted body fat due to complete amino acid insufficiency. Unfortunately, stored body fat produced from an overabundance of dietary protein cannot be reconverted back into amino acids. As with all food sources, too little or too much dietary protein is undesirable, but a diet containing just the right amount of balanced total protein will ensure optimum body redevelopment without the formation of unwanted body fat.

Choosing the right foods

Armed with the necessary understanding of body building proteins and their function, it is important to identify and choose reliable dietary sources of complete proteins. Most vegetable and grain proteins are lacking in some essential amino acids, especially lysine, tryptophan, threonine or methionine, and therefore cannot satisfactorily promote growth when consumed by themselves. Meat, fish, milk and egg protein, due to their complete amino acid composition and good digestibility, have a high biologic value and will satisfy the total needs of the human body.

Given the design of the human digestive system it is impossible for an individual to gain all of the protein necessary for optimum body development from vegetable sources alone. Herbivores consume incredible quantities of grass and leaves each day, spending the majority of their waking hours eating low energy carbohydrate foods. On average, an elephant in the wild will consume the foliage of 11 trees and a respectable intake of grass and shrubs each and every day of its life. An elephant will consume its entire body weight of approximately three to four tons every two weeks. Humans do not have the capacity to digest such quantities of vegetable matter. We eat on average for 40 minutes each day, and consume less than 2% of our body weight in food. Any diet devoid of con-centrated total protein from animal sources must therefore be deficient.

Herbivores also have the ability to digest and extract nutrients and protein from cellulose, the humanly indigestible part of fruit and vegetables we refer to as roughage or fibre. Although laboratory tests indicate a relatively high amino acid content in lentils, legumes and nuts, a good proportion of this protein is inextricably bound in the plants' cellulose structure. As the human digestive system lacks the ability to digest cellulose, these nutrients pass right on through our bodies.

Protein deficiency syndromes

Dietary protein deficiency syndromes are well known to science. Perhaps the most commonly apparent is kwashiorkor, a severe protein deficiency condition encountered in recent years in famine stricken Africa. Symptoms of severe protein malnutrition include diminished body development, fatigue, alterations to skin and hair pigmentation, fluid retention, liver and pancreatic damage, mental apathy, diarrhoea, anaemia, and retarded wound healing. Lesser deficiencies certainly yield milder symptoms, but the existence of this condition does demonstrate the absolute need for a constant supply of dietary protein for the maintenance of optimum health.

Former theories claiming excessive protein consumption may give rise to hypertension (high blood pressure), toxic complications during pregnancy, the encouragement of certain diseases, or the onset of liver and kidney damage have all been abandoned due to a total absence of credible scientific evidence. However, a diet consisting only of protein could give the body cause to degrade muscle and tissue for the production of essential glucose. This is a reactive function which may lead to the onset of the toxic and potentially fatal condition of ketosis.

It is apparent the daily intake of complete protein from concentrated sources such as red meat, fish, poultry, eggs and dairy products is essential to ensure adequate body repair and function. But, too little or too much protein, or diets advocating protein to the exclusion of carbohydrate and fats, are demonstrated health hazards.

CARBOHYDRATES

Carbohydrates are the sugars found in most fruit, vegetables and milk. The most common sugars are sucrose from sugar cane, glucose and fructose from fruit and honey, starch from vegetables and grains, and lactose from milk. Grouped according to physical structure, glucose and fructose are designated as simple carbohydrates or monosaccharides. Sucrose, lactose and starch are either disaccharides or polysaccharides and are members of the complex carbohydrate group. Irrespective of these classifications, all sugars are converted by the enzymes of the digestive tract into either glucose, fructose or galactose. The fructose and galactose are subsequently converted by the liver into glucose, which is the end product of all sugars entering the body. Consequently, the source of dietary carbohydrate is unimportant. The starch from a potato, the fructose from a piece of fruit, or the lactose from milk all end up as glucose once they enter the body. In addition to sugar, most carbohydrate foods of vegetable origin contain humanly non-digestible cellulose, some vitamins, minerals, a little incomplete protein and a lot of water.

How important is glucose?

Glucose plays a very important role in the production of body energy, however, its role has been grossly overemphasised. Any excess of carbohydrate to immediate energy requirements will be converted by the fat cells and the liver into triglycerides and stored as body fat. In consequence, sugar has become the western diet's single greatest contributor to stored body fat.

We generally refer to fruit, grains and vegetables as carbohydrates, but this may be misleading. The term carbohydrate is a derivation of carbon and hydrogen, the components of all sugars. Therefore, carbohydrate refers specifically to the sugar content of the food source and not to the food itself. It is more correct to refer to fruit, grains and vegetables as carbohydrate bearing foods, and not simply as carbohydrates. The carbohydrate content of each food source varies greatly, and this is a significant factor in choosing foods complementary to losing body fat, and keeping it off. For example, asparagus contains just 1% carbohydrate, but cane sugar is 100% pure carbohydrate. Therefore, a person could consume 100 times more asparagus by weight than pure cane sugar, and absorb the same amount of carbohydrate.

Two questionable assumptions of recent years have given rise to a massive increase in the overall consumption of dietary carbohydrate at the expense of essential proteins and fats. The first assumption erroneously identified carbohydrate as the primary energy source of the body. The second assumption quite wrongly labelled saturated fats as the prime contributors to elevated serum cholesterol levels. The resulting shift in dietary balance has had a negative effect on our bodies and our health, this has resulted in:

- the suppression of stored fat as an enduring energy source;
- the unprecedented elevation of serum cholesterol levels;
- a massive increase in the incidence of overweight and obesity; and
- an alarming elevation in the incidence of diagnosed diabetes.

Misconceptions regarding the intake of dietary fibre, vitamins and minerals have also had a profound effect on our overall consumption of carbohydrates. Carbohydrate foods eaten to excess may actually hinder the absorption of other essential nutrients and the passage of food through the system, adding to, rather than subtracting from, the problems of malnutrition and constipation.

How much carbohydrate is enough?

The inclusion of carbohydrate bearing foods in your daily diet is essential, but only in quantities calculated to supply your body with all of the vitamins, minerals, fibre and glucose necessary for non-fat forming good health. This you may achieve by limiting your intake of carbohydrates as suggested by your *Slim Forever* program, and confining your choices to the fresh fruit and vegetables appearing at the low end of the sugar content scale. A selection of nutritious, low carbohydrate, green and yellow vegetables should complement starchy foods such as potato, corn and rice. Fruit generally has a much higher sugar content than vegetables and in most cases is nutritionally inferior. Fruit grown commercially is usually picked green and held in storage at low temperatures before undergoing artificial ripening. This process denudes the product of much of its nutritional value. Make your choice based on freshness and the relative sugar content of each food source. And finally, avoid all manufactured or prepared foods containing highly concentrated cane or beet sugar.

By reducing your overall carbohydrate intake to correspond to your optimum daily carbohydrate allowance, your body will return to a normal level of function and you will lose that unwanted burden of fat. In time, your desire for sweeter foods will disappear to a point where they may become totally unappealing.

SATURATED AND UNSATURATED FATS

Fats are not only absolutely essential components of good nutrition, they may also be the most misunderstood ingredient in our diet.

Technically, the correct name for any fat or oil is lipid, but for ease of description we have labelled liquid lipids as oils, and solid lipids as fats. All lipids will liquefy when heated and solidify when refrigerated, but if a lipid is liquid at room temperature it is classified as an oil, and if it is solid it is a fat.

Lipids, be they oils or fats, are further classified according to their physical structure as being either saturated or unsaturated. Unsaturated lipids are further classified as being either mono-unsaturated or polyunsaturated depending upon each lipid's degree of unsaturation.

Lipids are chains of carbon atoms of varying lengths. Each carbon atom forming the chain has the ability to attach itself by means of atomic linkages to a maximum of two atoms of hydrogen. If all the carbon linkages are filled with hydrogen atoms, the lipid is said to be saturated, but if any linkages are left vacant, the lipid is classified as being unsaturated. One vacant link classifies a lipid as being mono-unsaturated, and two or more vacant links classify it as being polyunsaturated.

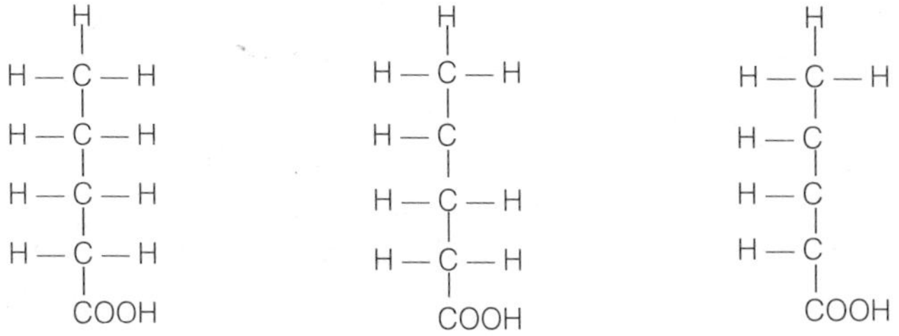

Saturated　　Mono-unsaturated　　Polyunsaturated

Configuration of Lipid Chains
Figure 9.1

Although the differences in saturation and chain length may appear insignificant, these differences are sufficient to give each individual fat its own particular character and role in human nutrition.

Why fats in the diet?

Dietary fats play many important roles in human physiological function. The principal function of fats is the supply of the body's most potent source of fuel for the production of energy and heat. Fats are essential for the absorption of vitamins A, D, E and K, and in the uptake and transport of bone and muscle building calcium. If ingested fat is not present in the intestine, these essential nutrients will not be absorbed into the bloodstream and will be passed out of the body on defecation.

Fats are essential ingredients in the development of nerves, skin, and some hormones, and deposited fat forms a protective shock absorbing layer around certain organs. The wide distribution of fat over the surface of the body acts as a thermal shield against outside cold. Fats supply the only useable form of energy to heart muscle, the very same organ we are supposedly protecting by eliminating fats from our diet.

Fats also play important roles in sexual maturation, pregnancy and the production of milk in the lactating female. One very positive effect of dietary fat is the control it exerts over the hunger response. Fat takes up to 3½ hours to clear from the stomach prior to commencing its journey along the intestinal tract, a delay instrumental in actively reducing perceived hunger.

The downside to eliminating fats from the diet

The effects of eliminating fats from our diet are now clearly evident. Clinically detectible problems such as joint pain, insatiable hunger, diminished immune response, impaired nutrient uptake, dry skin and deformed nail growth have been reported in humans. Laboratory rats fed fat-free diets produced the specific problems of retarded body growth, scaly skin, kidney failure and early death.

Saturated and unsaturated fats differ only slightly in composition. Both are constructed largely of triglycerides, and each contains small amounts of essential phospholipids and sterols, and in some cases vitamins A and D. Saturated animal fats contain small amounts of cholesterol which, contrary to popular propaganda, is a compound of great physiological importance.

Essential fatty acids

Unsaturated fats are cholesterol free, and they do contain linoleic, linolenic and arachidonic fatty acids not found in saturated fats. Known as the essential fatty acids, the need for their presence in the diet is well documented.

Essential fatty acids are so named because of their essential roles in the structural development of cell membranes, the promotion of blood clotting and the manufacture of essential prostaglandins. Although an understanding of the role of prostaglandins is relatively new, these hormone-like substances are now known to positively influence life at the cellular level. Any decrease in the dietary uptake of essential fatty acids may lead to a suppression of prostaglandin production and the possible onset of cardiovascular disease, stroke, elevated blood pressure, infection, sexual dysfunction, cancer, eczema and psoriasis of the skin, arthritis, schizophrenia, depression and hyperactivity (Gittleman, A.L., *Beyond Pritikin,* 1989).

Trans-fatty acids

The production of prostaglandins hangs in a delicate balance. Fatty acids occur naturally as cis-fatty acids, but these healthy fats can be converted into a toxic form of fat known as trans-fatty acids by the application of excessive heat. Commercial cooking oil, and its by-products margarine and vegetable shortening, are manufactured using extremely high levels of heat. In consequence, all products made from heat extracted oils contain a large percentage of trans-fatty acids. Once in the bloodstream these humanly toxic trans-fatty acids compete with the healthy cis-fatty acids, effectively blocking prostaglandin production, weakening cell membranes and reducing resistance to disease.

In recent years, saturated fats of animal origin have been branded the bad guys, and unsaturated oils from vegetable sources hailed as the good guys. But, generally classifying animal fats as being saturated and vegetable fats as being unsaturated is incorrect. It is rare to find a fat of any description that is either totally saturated, or totally unsaturated. This is clearly demonstrated by the following chart (Table 9.1).

FOOD SOURCE	% SATURATED FAT TO TOTAL FAT	% UNSATURATED FAT TO TOTAL FAT
Pork- lean	33	67
- with fat	42	58
Chicken - with skin	25	75
- flesh only	33	67
Steak - lean	50	50
- with fat	50	50
Eggs	40	60
Cheese, cheddar	60	40
Cream, whipping	60	40
Milk, whole cream	63	37
Coconut	93	7
Peanuts	24	76
Avocados	39	61
Butter	60	40
Margarine	24	76
Olive oil	14	86
Corn oil	8	92
Soybean oil	17	83

Fat Content of Various Foods
Table 9.1

Source: Figures derived from United States Department of Agriculture, 'Nutritive values of the edible parts of foods', *Home and Garden Bulletin* No.72, Washington D.C., 1970.

Of all the food sources appearing in Table 9.1, oil extracted from coconuts is the most saturated fat known, yet it is a vegetable oil used widely in the production of commercial frying oils and vegetable shortening. Not only is extracted coconut oil highly saturated, it also contains trans-fatty acids, a legacy of the high heat employed in the extraction process. It has become fashionable for commercial enterprises serving deep-fried food to advertise the use of pure vegetable oils in the frying process. But, if those oils happen to contain coconut or palm oils, the product they use may well be more saturated than beef fat.

An optimum ratio of saturated fats to unsaturated fats in the human diet has not been established, but given a diet with a balance of all the major food groups, any such determination may be unnecessary. The unsaturated fat content of the essential protein sources of beef, pork, poultry and eggs ranges from 50% to 75% of total fat depending on the food source. This ratio of unsaturated fats to saturated fats is more than sufficient to satisfy our essential fatty acid requirements.

Chemical and heat damaged oils

Our bodies are not at odds with the natural fats we eat, but rather with the processed and radically altered fats currently invading our food chain. The excessive heat and chemicals used in the extraction of vegetable oils has created a health problem of enormous proportions.

The first edible oil of vegetable origin was from olives and was extracted by physically crushing the olives at room temperature and squeezing the oil out. Used in cooking and in the making of salad dressings, the popularity of olive oil grew, and the demand saw oils extracted from sources such as safflower, corn and peanuts soon became commercially available.

Early methods of oil extraction were crude and wasteful with much of the oil content being discarded along with the pulp. Science came to the rescue and added heat in the range of 250°F/120°C to the extraction process. The rate of recovery of the oil content increased considerably, but still a measure of oil remained untapped. Hexane, a close relative of gasoline and an irritant to the nervous system in humans, was added to the process and the last drops of oil were retrieved.

The efficiency of this process allowed vegetable oils to be produced at a fraction of the previous cost, but there were other problems to be overcome. Free fatty acids in the oil cause it to become cloudy, and these are removed by the addition of caustic soda and again heating the oil to 170°F/75°C. To remove the remnants of the hexane and caustic soda, the temperature of the oil is reduced and water and phosphoric acid are added. This process also removes the nutrients lecithin, acetylcholine and chlorophyll which would otherwise attract oxygen and cause the oil to spoil. The minerals calcium, magnesium, iron and copper are also removed.

Extracted oil is dark in colour which proved unappealing to the buying public. Not to be outdone, the oil manufacturing industry developed a method of bleaching the unwanted pigments in the oil. This is achieved by reheating the oil to 230°F/110°C and passing the oil through Fuller's earth or clay filters. This also removes the nutrient beta-carotene which the body converts into vitamin A. At this point in the refinement process toxic peroxides begin to form in the oil. Peroxides cause a cross-linking of the fatty acid chains which produces unnatural mutations and the formation of hybrid fats.

Vegetable oil has a distinctive and rather pungent odour which also proved unappealing to the buying public. The oil is deodorised by distilling it with steam at high temperatures for a period of one hour. Many of the remaining healthy cis-fatty acids which had previously resisted the application of heat now succumb and form toxic trans-fatty acids.

At some point during the refining process of unsaturated oils natures own preservative, vitamin E, is removed. This leaves the oil extremely susceptible to bacterial and fungal infestation. These marketing problems are overcome by the addition of yet more chemicals such as benzoic acid (used to season tobacco, and in the manufacture of toothpaste and germicides) and sodium benzoate (used as a food preservative and in the manufacture of antiseptic, commercial dyes and pharmaceuticals).

To preserve the oil against any form of spoilage, and to guarantee long shelflife, chemicals such as butyl-hydroxyanisole (BHA) and butyl-hydroxytoluene (BHT) are added. Both BHA and BHT are suspected cancer forming agents in humans. The preservatives gum guaiac, propyl gallate, gallic acid and ascorbic acid may also be used.

By comparison, the combination of saturated and unsaturated fats from animal sources are more stable when exposed to the air. The retention of natural preservatives attributes to the natural resistance of fresh fats to oxidation and rancidity.

Hydrogenation

As most vegetable oils are liquid at room temperature they are not suitable for the production of margarine or vegetable shortening. This obstacle is overcome by again heating the oil and adding hydrogen gas and nickel. Nickel is used in the industrial manufacture of alloys, car batteries and in the electroplating of metal. It is also a known carcinogen in humans. Activated by heat, the nickel reacts with the unsaturated carbon atoms of the fatty acid chains to attract molecules of hydrogen in a process known as hydrogenation. By comparison, animal fats are a combination of natural and relatively stable saturated and unsaturated fats. But, the devitalised and lifeless plastic oils produced by the process of refinement and hydrogenation become highly saturated.

THE GREAT MARGARINE DECEPTION

The degree of artificial saturation by hydrogenation determines the hardness of the finished product. Highly saturated vegetable oils are extremely hard and ideal for use in the manufacture of vegetable shortening, but total saturation makes the product too hard for the manufacture of margarine. The degree of saturation in oils used in the manufacture of margarine is controlled by limiting the saturation process to produce a product which is easy to spread. Or alternatively, by fully saturating the oil and then adding back liquid oil until the degree of desired product softness is achieved. In any event the level of unnatural trans-fatty acids produced by the refinement and hydrogenation processes can be as high as 47% of the total fat content. A number of countries have legislated to limit the trans-fatty acid content in refined foods to around 1% by volume. The Dutch legislated a 0% trans-fatty acid content which meant an immediate ban on the sale of margarine and other refined oil products in that country.

The oils used in the manufacture of vegetable shortening and margarine may have been polyunsaturated at one time, but that was long ago in the manufacturing process. Statistics available for the United States indicate approximately five million tons of damaged hydrogenated fats are consumed annually. A good percentage of these damaged fats is consumed as margarine, a product released onto the market at the end of the Second World War.

The history of margarine

The name margarine is a derivation of two words — margar from margaric, meaning pearl; and ine meaning made of or resembling. The chosen name accurately described the pearly white colour of the original product, but the colour failed to attract the attention of the buying public. In the early 1950s a yellow colouring was added to bring it closer in appearance to its arch rival, butter.

Before elevated serum cholesterol levels became medically fashionable, margarine was marketed on its physical characteristic of being easily spread when taken directly from the refrigerator. The current thrust of margarine advertising is directed at the cholesterol free market with the express message that cholesterol free vegetable oils are good for your health, and animal fats are bad.

The labels on many margarine containers inform us that the product is vitamin enriched. Vitamins A and D are added presumably to offset the nutritional damage done to the natural oils during processing. Vitamin A occurs naturally in liver, kidney, cream, butter, egg yolks and in green and yellow vegetables. Vitamin D is only found in yeast and fish liver oils. The vitamin enrichment process does nothing to replace the 19 naturally occuring vitamins and minerals lost during manufacture.

The truth about margarine

In the final analysis the product known as margarine may well be described as a cocktail of damaged and nutritionally denuded supersaturated oils, high in destructive trans-fatty acids and added toxic chemicals.

In an act of complete deception the manufacturers of vegetable oils, margarine and vegetable shortening gather the nutritional information appearing on the label from fresh squeezed oils, not from the oils contained in the finished product (Erdmann, R. and Jones, M., *Fats Nutrition and Health*, 1990).

A new product has made its way onto our supermarket shelves in recent years. To capture the buyers who want the best of all worlds, a combination of butter and vegetable oil is being offered. This product may best be described as the good, the bad and the ugly.

THE GOOD OIL ON FATS

Like butter? Butter is a cold processed, nutritionally intact and natural derivative of milk, with only one strike against it.

The manufacturers add potassium chloride (widely used in the manufacture of some fertiliser) as a preservative. Dr Erdmann and Meirion Jones describe butter as being "not only highly nutritious but an underexposed form of alternative health therapy".

The problem with fat consumption is not with the fats we can see, but rather with the fats we cannot see. We have taken to removing most of the fresh and naturally vital fats from the food we eat in favour of eating enormous quantities of damaged toxic fats. Nutritionally damaged, supersaturated, hydrogenated and chemically polluted fats are widely used in the manufacture of processed foods, significantly increasing the percentage of saturated fats we consume. This increase in unnatural, damaged saturated fats over healthy saturated and unsaturated fats poses a threat to the health of every person who eats them.

Mono-unsaturated oils such as olive, peanut and avocado oils are more stable than are the polyunsaturated oils. Tests indicate that oils made from these sources better complement ingested saturated fats. Unfortunately peanut oil is often heat extracted, and avocado oil is expensive, but olive oil is cold pressed and nutrient retentive, and is an excellent oil for salad dressings. However, even cold pressed mono-unsaturated oils will form some trans-fatty acids when used for frying, which does not happen with butter.

How much fat is enough?

A rule of thumb when consuming fats is to trim the visible fat from meat prior to cooking to a maximum of $\frac{1}{8}$ in/3 mm of the lean flesh. Broil or grill your food where possible and let any excess fat drain away. Skim floating fat from stews, braises and casseroles before serving, and use butter, never margarine. Restrict or avoid completely all fast foods cooked in oil and precooked frozen dinners, and make your salad dressings from scratch using cold pressed olive, avocado or peanut oils.

Fresh, unspoiled and non-toxic saturated and unsaturated fats play an important and essential biological role in the human body. As is the case with proteins and carbohydrates, the quality and quantity of the ingested fats you eat is important, but under no circumstances should fresh fats be omitted from your diet.

10

vitamins and minerals

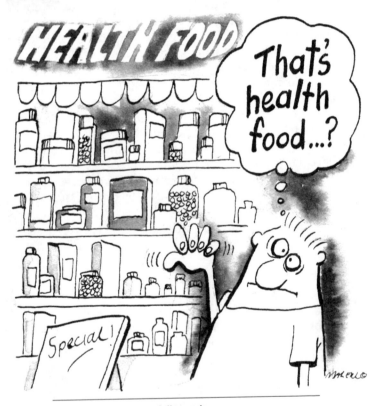

VITAMINS

Vitamins were the last group of dietary essentials to be recognised. This is easy to understand, since they are needed in such very small amounts.

Dr Helen Andrews Guthrie, 1975

Vitamins constitute a group of dietetically essential organic substances necessary to human metabolic function, but, due to the low concentration of vitamins in all food sources, their discovery was overlooked until the beginning of the twentieth century. The general classification in 1912 of these nutrients as vitamins is credited to Casimir Funk, a Polish-born biochemist employed at the Lister Institute in London. He coined the name *vitamine* for the Greek *vita* meaning life, and *amine*, derived from the mistaken identification of many of these substances as belonging to the amine group. The *e* was later dropped as many of the vitamins proved not to be amines at all.

The discovery of the various vitamins was spread over a period of 33 years from 1915 to 1948, and as each of the early discoveries was made it was labelled with a letter of the alphabet. The alphabetising of the vitamins was largely a failure as gaps soon appeared when certain substances were later found not to be vitamins at all, or in some cases were vitamins already discovered and previously named. As an understanding of the structure of vitamins progressed, certain vitamins were grouped together and renamed, but still within the alphabetical naming structure. For instance, similarities were discovered between vitamin B and vitamin G, and these were subsequently renamed vitamin B_1 and vitamin B_2 respectively. The space originally occupied by vitamin G became vacant and has not been reused.

The current trend is to replace the alphabetised names of these substances with their generic names. For instance, by common usage vitamin C is becoming more broadly referred to by its generic name of ascorbic acid, and vitamin B_1 as thiamine, and so on. In time we may cease using the alphabetic coding system altogether.

The early discovery of vitamins was largely due to efforts in seeking the mysterious missing factors in a number of presenting diseases. Funk's original discovery followed a change he made in the diet of his pet pigeons from rice bran to polished rice. His pet birds developed weakness of body movement due to nerve impairment, commonly referred to as beriberi. Although Funk did not isolate the mystery factor necessary to prevent beriberi, he was able to deduce it was present in rice bran but not present in polished rice. This confirmed the theory that disease could be related to dietary inadequacy of certain factors in food, which he generally referred to as vitamines.

It took another 24 years of intensive research before the mystery substance thiamine (vitamin B_1) was isolated as the anti-beriberi factor. Similarly, ascorbic acid (vitamin C) inadequacy was subsequently linked to the deadly sailors' disease of scurvy. Cobalamin (vitamin B_{12}) was found to be the missing ingredient in pernicious anaemia, and niacin with pellagra, a disease associated with the corn dominant diets of southern Europeans. The last vitamin to be discovered was cobalamin (vitamin B_{12}) in 1948, but the book on vitamins cannot yet be closed as the possibility of discovery of other as yet unknown factors cannot be dismissed.

Vitamins are classified as being either fat soluble or water soluble. The fat soluble vitamins A, D, E and K are not water soluble and can only be absorbed into the body in the presence of dietary fats. The remaining 11 vitamins are all water soluble.

The need for vitamins among the various species in the animal kingdom varies considerably. For example, vitamin C must be supplied in the diet to humans, primates and guinea pigs, but it is synthesised by the body in many other species including rats, rabbits and dogs. The human body can synthesise certain vitamins from substances which are not themselves vitamins but are close chemical relatives of certain specific vitamins. These are referred to as pro-vitamins. For instance, the intestine can synthesise retinol (vitamin A) from carotene in the diet, and the kidneys can synthesise cholecalciferol (vitamin D) from 7–dehydrocholesterol, a substance produced by the activity of the sun's rays on the skin.

Vitamins perform no direct function in the human body. Vitamins are coenzymes which act as catalysts to the initiation of function of specific enzymes. Each living cell contains greater than 500 specific nonactivated enzymes, some of which can initiate metabolic activity without help. Others, however, require the assistance of specific vitamins to become activated. The presence of a vitamin specific to a particular enzyme is so critical that if the vitamin is not available in the bloodstream at the precise moment of metabolic activity, the entire process will abort.

Vitamin deficiencies may arise for a number of reasons. Poor storage and preparation of fresh foods and damaging production methods employed by commercial food manufacturers will substantially reduce vitamin levels in food even before we get to eat it. Dietary imbalance and overeating are also major contributing factors. Failure to consume foods specific in the supply of all of the necessary vitamins will adversely affect vitamin balance, and the absence of fats in the diet will preclude the absorption of the fat soluble vitamins, a common failing with vegetarian diets.

It would be reasonable to assume the more a person eats the greater will be the volume of absorbed vitamins and other nutrients, but this is not necessarily the case. When food is consumed to excess, the rate of travel of the food through the intestine is accelerated, and the sheer bulk makes it impossible for much of the food to make contact with the absorptive surface of the intestine. A combination of massive eating and nutritionally poor food, often results in many big eaters becoming malnourished and overweight.

Table 10.1 lists the vitamins under their respective classifications of being either fat soluble or water soluble; their principal actions within the body; and their primary food sources in descending order of concentration.

VITAMIN	ACTION WITHIN THE BODY	PRIMARY FOOD SOURCES
Fat soluble vitamins		
Retinol (vitamin A)	Night vision DNA synthesis Cellular construction Tissue growth Fertility	Liver Eggs Milk Cheese Butter
Cholecalciferol (vitamin D)	Bone calcification Protein stability	Sunshine Eggs Milk Butter Fish oils

Tocopherol (vitamin E)	Anti-toxicant
	Cellular respiration
	Haemoglobin formation
	Cell membrane structure
		Wheat germ,
		  corn, soybean
		  cottonseed &
		  safflower oils
		Beef liver
		Butter

Phytylmenaquinone (vitamin K)	Blood coagulation	Green & yellow vegetables Alfalfa Dairy products Eggs Liver
Water soluble vitamins		
Thiamine (vitamin B_1)	Carbohydrate metabolism Protein synthesis High frequency nerve transmission	Wheat germ Pecans & peanuts Pork Legumes Eggs Beef

Riboflavin (vitamin B_2)	Energy production
	Protein metabolism
	Corticosteroid
	  production
	Red blood cell
	  formation
	Thyroid activity
		Dairy products
		Red meat
		Fish
		Poultry
		Eggs
		Grain cereals

VITAMIN	ACTION WITHIN THE BODY	PRIMARY FOOD SOURCES
Pantothenic acid (vitamin B_3)	Energy release Fat synthesis Nerve transmission Drug anti-toxicant Antibody stimulation Cholesterol synthesis Absorption of glucose	Liver Egg yolk Kidney Wheat bran Broccoli Lima beans Beef Milk products
Pyridoxine (vitamin B_6)	Protein, carbohydrate & fat metabolism Cerebral activity Haemoglobin synthesis Antibody production	Red meat Fish Poultry Eggs Bananas Cabbage Lima Beans Potatoes Dairy products
Cobalamin (vitamin B_{12})	Anti-anaemia factor Blood formation Body growth Maintenance of nervous tissue Carbohydrate, protein & fat metabolism	Liver Oysters All meats Eggs Fish & shrimp Dairy products
Ascorbic Acid (vitamin C)	Formation of collagen, scar tissue & tooth enamel Iron & calcium uptake Folic acid activation Adrenal hormone secretion	Green peppers Broccoli Leafy vegetables Strawberries Citrus fruit Tomatoes Liver
Biotin (vitamin H)	Carbon dioxide removal Protein synthesis Fat & carbohydrate metabolism	Liver & kidney Milk Egg yolk Yeast Cauliflower Nuts Legumes
Folacin (vitamin M)	Cell proliferation Amino acid synthesis	Pork liver Asparagus Kidney beans Carrots Beef Potatoes Dairy products Chicken

VITAMIN	ACTION WITHIN THE BODY	PRIMARY FOOD SOURCES
Niacin	Energy production DNA formation Nutrient utilisation	Red meat Fish Poultry Eggs Oranges Spinach
Choline	Liver fat mobilisation Nerve transmission	Egg yolk Beef liver Soybeans Fish Grain cereals

Inositol	Liver & bone marrow
	  growth
	Heart, brain & muscle
	  function
		All meats
		Milk
		Fruit
		Nuts
		Vegetables
		Grain cereals

Vitamin Activity and Source
Table 10.1

A widely held misconception suggests fruit and vegetables are the major source of dietary vitamins, but this is certainly not the case. Of the 15 known vitamins only three are primarily or exclusively derived from plant sources, while the remaining 12 vitamins are derived either primarily or exclusively from animal products.

Just what quantity of vitamins we should consume is a point of contention. Various committees, including the World Health Organization, suggest varying levels of daily vitamin intake, but the recommended daily requirements of any vitamin must be considered to be arbitrary. Firstly, the normal daily requirements of specific vitamins can vary fourfold between individuals. Therefore, if the greater requirement is accepted as being the minimum daily requirement, the majority of people could be consuming these vitamins to excess. Secondly, the greater requirement by an individual for a particular vitamin does not necessarily herald a need for an increase in all other vitamins for the same individual. In establishing the quantitative need for vitamins, other factors such as the general health of the individual, diet, stress, smoking, alcohol consumption and daily exercise level must be considered. Notwithstanding, and with the exception of cases involving specific and proven vitamin deficiencies, a balanced diet will supply more than adequate supplies of all of the vitamins necessary for good health.

The under consumption of vitamins can have obvious repercussions, but so too can the over supply of vitamins, especially those in the fat soluble group. Water soluble vitamins consumed to excess display greater propensity for eradication in the urine, a trait not shared by the fat soluble vitamins. The over consumption of any vitamin can lead to a condition known as hypervitaminosis, which becomes symptomatic according to the particular vitamin involved. For instance, the excessive consumption of non-dietary retinol (vitamin A) can produce the symptoms of headache, drowsiness, nausea, loss of hair, dry and scaly skin, weight loss, anorexia, skeletal pain in infants, diarrhoea in adults and the cessation of menstruation in females. Other vitamins consumed to excess exhibit different symptoms. However, it is fortunate the effects of hypervitaminosis will usually undergo rapid reversal following a decrease in dosage.

There does exist yet another variety of hypervitaminosis. Over zealous expectant mothers who take large doses of vitamins such as ascorbic acid (vitamin C) often give birth to babies with greater than normal requirements of those particular vitamins. As a result, the new born may subsequently exhibit symptoms of deficiency following restricted postnatal vitamin intake.

MINERALS

Approximately 4% of total body weight, about 6 lb/2.75 kg in the average adult male, is comprised of 60 or so mineral elements. Twenty-one of these elements have been proven essential to human nutrition.

Unlike the water soluble vitamins which can largely be flushed from the body if consumed to excess, minerals tend to remain in the body. The body can tolerate excesses of some minerals without the onset of toxicity, but with other minerals such as zinc, iron, cobalt, copper and selenium the level of intake must remain within a very specific and limited range. Insufficient intake of these minerals may give rise to the onset of disease, while minerals consumed to excess could lead to the onset of blood toxicity.

The 21 mineral elements considered essential to good health are divided into two groups. The minerals comprising the first designated group in Table 10.2 have been labelled macronutrients as these are the essential minerals found in the greatest concentration in the human body. The second group comprises the micronutrient minerals which are also essential to life, but which are found in lesser concentration in the body. The third group of minerals shows evidence of biological essentiality, but their roles are not yet conclusively proven. This group is referred to collectively as the probable nutrients. The fourth group of non-nutrients are the minerals found in the human body for which no metabolic role has been established. Some of the elements listed in this group are considered toxic to humans, and their number continues to grow as we absorb yet more commercially produced chemicals into our systems.

GROUP I (Macronutrients)	GROUP II (Micronutrients)	GROUP III (Probable nutrients)	GROUP IV (Non-nutrients)
Calcium	Iron	Barium	Gold
Phosphorus	Zinc	Arsenic	Silver
Potassium	Selenium	Bromine	Aluminium
Sulphur	Manganese	Strontium	Mercury
Chlorine	Copper	Cadmium	Bismuth
Magnesium	Iodine		Gallium
	Molybdenum		Lead
	Cobalt		Antimony
	Chromium		Boron
	Fluorine		Lithium
	Silicon		
	Vanadium		
	Nickel		
	Tin		

Mineral Nutrient Groups
Table 10.2

Like the vitamins, minerals act as catalysts for many metabolic reactions in our bodies. These reactions include the absorption and utilisation of proteins, fats and carbohydrates, and the production of energy. The formation of haemoglobin and the clotting of blood are also mineral dependant, as is the active transport of many nutrients from the bloodstream to the cells.

Minerals act as catalysts in the synthesis of many hormones, enzymes, and essential acids, and may form part of the finished products. Minerals are the essential ingredients in maintaining water balance in the kidneys, without which we would either dehydrate or drown in our own body fluids. The minerals we consume in our food also play major roles in the transmission of nerve impulses, in the process of muscle contraction and relaxation, and in essential body growth.

Table 10.3 indicates the function and primary food sources in order of greatest concentration of the major minerals found in the human body.

MINERAL	ACTION WITHIN THE BODY	PRIMARY FOOD SOURCES
Calcium	Bone & tooth formation Body growth Blood clotting Biological catalyst Cell membrane function Muscle contraction	Dairy products Fruit & vegetables Grain cereals & beans All meats Eggs Fats & oils
Phosphorus	Energy regulation Nutrient transportation Enzyme & DNA composition Calcification of bones & teeth Acid–base regulation	All meats Fish Eggs Dairy products Peas Lima beans
Potassium	Energy release Protein synthesis Fluid pressure Nerve transmission Insulin release	Avocado Apricots Bananas All meats Fish Potato
Sulphur	Cell, hair, skin & nail formation Blood clotting Detoxifying agent Collagen synthesis	All meats

MINERAL	ACTION WITHIN THE BODY	PRIMARY FOOD SOURCES
Sodium	Fluid pressure Water balance Acid–base regulation Nerve transmission Glucose absorption	Salt-added foods Eggs Celery Chicken Milk Carrots
Chlorine	Cerebrospinal fluid Gastric secretions Acid–base regulation Carbon dioxide transportation	Common salt
Magnesium	Major biological catalyst Energy production Nutrient absorption & transportation Cellular respiration Amino acid utilisation Muscle relaxation	Nuts Soybeans Grain cereals Spinach Crustaceans All meats Eggs Most fruit & vegetables
Iron	Oxygen carrier Blood formation Vitamin A formation Blood fat eradication Antibody production Drug detoxification Breast milk antibodies	Pork, lamb, calf, beef & chicken liver All meats Fish Eggs Grain cereals Fruit & vegetables
Iodine	Thyroxine formation	Crustaceans Saltwater fish Drinking water Dairy products Eggs Spinach Iodised table salt
Zinc	Body growth Sexual maturity Wound healing	Oysters, shrimp & tuna All meats Peanuts Dairy products Eggs Grain cereals Leafy vegetables Legumes

MINERAL	ACTION WITHIN THE BODY	PRIMARY FOOD SOURCES
Manganese	Tissue growth Synthesis of fats & cholesterol Liver fat release Energy release	Grain cereals Nuts Legumes Tea Leafy vegetables All meats Dairy products Seafood
Copper	Anaemia prevention Phospholipid synthesis Melanin production	Liver Shellfish Nuts Mushrooms Grain cereals Leafy vegetables All meats
Molybdenum	Mobilisation of liver iron reserves Dental decay inhibitor	Legumes All meats Grain cereals
Selenium	Anti-toxicant Cancer growth retardant	Seafood All meats Grain cereals
Chromium	Glucose utilisation Insulin activity	Most vegetables Grain cereals Fruit
Cobalt	Anti-anaemia agent Some enzyme activity	Liver All meats Saltwater fish Milk
Silicon	Bone formation	Milk Animal products Fruit & vegetables
Tin	Body tissue growth Wound healing Protein synthesis Energy metabolism	All meats Grain cereals Legumes Fruit & vegetables
Vanadium	Body tissue, bone & tooth formation	Grain cereals Root vegetables Nuts
Fluorine	Control of tooth decay Body tissue growth	Tea & coffee Rice Soybeans Spinach Onions

Mineral Activity and Source
Table 10.3

VITAMIN AND MINERAL REQUIREMENTS

The human need for vitamins and minerals, while being absolutely essential to life, remains extremely small. We developed as a species in harmony with our environment, and we are in fact an extension of that environment. The basic components of our bodies are an assortment of minerals in their various forms from the earth and the oceans of our planet. Had our need for nutrients been greater than the planet was able to supply in our food chain, we would not have survived.

In evaluating the optimum level of vitamin and mineral intake, it is important we do not fall into the trap of believing that if a given quantity of any vitamin or mineral is essential for good health, a larger quantity will necessarily be better. Vitamins and minerals either assist, or enter into, a huge assortment of metabolic functions within our bodies, but they do not initiate those functions. No amount of ingested vitamins or minerals will initiate new function or extend the duration of any function beyond the limits imposed by our bodies.

Once absorbed into the body the vitamins and minerals enter a metabolic pool, there to await functional selection. The capacity of the metabolic pool is not large simply because our daily consumption of vitamins and minerals is quite small. For example, below is the National Research Council of the United States' recommended daily allowance of retinol (vitamin A) in international units (IU) and the equivalent in both ounces and grams:

For the adult male: 5000 IU or $\frac{1}{2500}$ oz/$\frac{1}{900}$ g.

For the adult female: 4000 IU or $\frac{1}{3500}$ oz/$\frac{1}{1125}$ g.

Therefore, the recommended daily allowance of retinol is available, for example, from:

- ■ $\frac{1}{4}$ cup of spinach or carrots; or
- ■ $\frac{1}{3}$ oz/9 g of beef liver.

As is the case with all vitamins and minerals, our daily food chain contains many times the recommended daily allowance.

Our need for essential vitamins and minerals has been grossly exaggerated. An entire industry has been established based on the manufacture and sale of vitamin and mineral pills of every imaginable combination. Using the metabolic function of a vitamin or mineral as a basis, the manufacturers make medicine-man-like claims as to the positive effects these various concoctions will have on our bodies. It is sad, but true, that those who take a daily vitamin and mineral supplement usually have no advantage over those who don't, other than to have more expensive urine.

Our bodies have changed little during recent millennia, and a diet balanced in proteins, fats and carbohydrates to include red meat, liver, poultry, seafood, dairy products and a selection of fruit and vegetables such as green peppers, broccoli, spinach, squash, pumpkin, carrot, lettuce, avocado, tomato, potato and banana will supply the human body with an abundance of all of the life giving vitamins and minerals.

It is interesting to note that the fruit and vegetables highest in vitamins and minerals are also those with the lowest carbohydrate content, and are the least fattening.

ACID-BASE BALANCE

Just as the body functions best at a specific level of temperature control, so too does it function best at a point of balance between acids and alkalies. This is referred to as the acid-base balance.

Most of us judge the relative levels of acidity or alkalinity of the foods we eat by the perceived level of acidity on our taste buds. As confusing as it may seem, the amount of acid present in a food is irrelevant. The acid forming properties of food are not determined by the amount of acid it contains, but rather by the components of the non-combustible mineral ash it contains. If the mineral ash contains chlorine, sulphur or phosphorus the action on the body will be acidic, but if the food contains calcium, sodium, potassium or magnesium the action will be alkaline. These elements may of course coexist in the same food source, but as they become separated during digestion, each specific element will exert its own influence on the acid-base balance.

Contrary to popular belief, the acid forming foods are the protein foods such as red meat, poultry, fish and eggs. The alkaline forming foods include most fruit and vegetables. The acids we detect in fruit, such as citric acid in oranges, does not have the opportunity to act as an acid. Once it enters the body it is immediately broken down to form carbon dioxide, water and energy. The energy is used by the body, and the carbon dioxide and water are respectively eradicated during exhalation and urination.

Some foods, such as cranberries, rhubarb, cocoa and tea, break this rule as they contain acids such as benzoic acid, oxalic acid and tannic acid which the body is unable to metabolise. When ingested, these unaltered acids will negatively influence the acid-base balance.

The body protects the acid-base balance by releasing carbonates, phosphates and proteins to neutralise the excesses of both acids and alkalies. If these soft balancing agents fail to maintain equilibrium, the body will produce nitrous hydroxide to neutralise any excess of acid, or carbonic acid to neutralise alkali excesses. Dietary imbalance due to vegetarianism, extremely high intakes of protein to the exclusion of carbohydrate, or the prolonged use of antacids, will each severely tax the body's ability to maintain acid-base neutrality.

COMMON SALT

The need for salt in the diet has become a matter of contention. Salts exist in many forms, most of which are toxic to the human body, but the salt we refer to as common or table salt is sodium chloride ($NaCl$), a very important human mineral source.

Ingested common salt does not stay in its predigested state once it enters the body. Once consumed, salt is broken down into its constituent parts of sodium (Na) and chloride (Cl) during the digestion process. Sodium, one of the more plentiful of the minerals in the human body, is necessary in the maintenance of internal water balance and pressure, and contributes to the balance between acids and alkalies. It exerts control over each cell's ability to absorb nutrients, and glucose, and plays an important role in the transmission or nerve impulses to contracting muscles. Chloride plays a similar role to sodium in maintaining both the water and the acid-base balance. It singularly contributes to the production of hydrochloric acid (HCl) in the stomach which is an acid necessary for the predigestion of the food we eat. The nutrient rich cerebrospinal fluid surrounding the brain and spinal cord is especially rich in chloride.

Sodium and chloride are both readily absorbed by the body and their balance is under the control of the kidneys. Any excess to daily requirements of either sodium or chloride is discharged into the urine and excreted from the body. Sources of dietary sodium are table salt, milk and meat, but chloride is only found in any appreciable quantity in table salt.

The loss of these essential salts through excessively perspiring, vomiting or having diarrhoea can lead to general body weakness, fatigue, lack of appetite, nausea and a reduction in mental acuity. Kidney malfunction may occur in cases of severe salt deficiency. People who work in intense heat usually add salt to their drinking water to replace salt lost as a result of perspiring. Ironically, body deficiencies of sodium and chloride will give rise to unquenchable thirst, a thirst capable of being alleviated only by the administration of salt, not fluid. In the extreme, tests involving rats showed severe salt deficiencies give rise to retardation of growth, muscle wasting, atrophy of the testes in the male, and degeneration of living tissue.

As with all dietary considerations, too much may be as damaging as too little, and salt is no exception. There is credible evidence supporting a relationship between excessive salt intake and chronic hypertension (elevated blood pressure). But, the damage done to our bodies by excessive salt intake may not necessarily be attributable just to the essential minerals, sodium and chloride. The salt we buy in the supermarket is largely mined from deposits left behind by the drying up of sea beds, in many cases millions of years ago. Originally these salt deposits were pure sodium chloride, but over time the seeping rains have carried with them many other humanly toxic minerals. As the rains soaked down through the salt beds, the toxic mineral salts were absorbed into the mass deposits of sodium chloride, and these too end up in our food.

The good news is that salt extracted directly from the sea is pure sodium chloride, and is available in health food stores and some supermarkets. Unfortunately, sea salt is less than snow white, and tends to absorb water. To overcome these traits many manufacturers add chemical bleaching and water retardant agents to their product to make it more appealing to the consumer. However, virgin salt is available.

Some researchers have suggested that sodium and chloride can be derived in sufficient quantities from the vegetables in our diet, while others oppose this view. The presence of common salt in our diets in the form of pure sodium chloride is essential, be it contained within the food, or added. Notwithstanding, the addition of salt to our food must be done in moderation as table salt can be addictive. The more salt you add to your food the more salt you will desire, so practise using it sparingly.

The wholesale addition of preservatives to manufactured food may be the real villains in the salt debate. These preservatives are all mineral salts, but they are all toxic salts, and they may play a greater role in hypertension and arterial wall damage than is currently apparent.

Due to its availability and cost, mined salt is predominantly chosen over sea salt in the manufacture of processed food, and is often added in abnormally high quantities. It is not necessarily the quantity of the salt we knowingly add to our food, but rather the unseen salt added during the manufacture of processed food that does the damage.

Sea salt is milder to the taste and consequently less addictive than mined salt. To balance your salt intake, restrict or eliminate processed foods from your diet, and add sea salt to your cooking and prepared food in moderation. As with all food sources, sodium and chloride are essential to the life process, but too little or too much will interfere with the natural balance and function of your body.

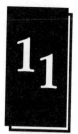

11

all about body fat

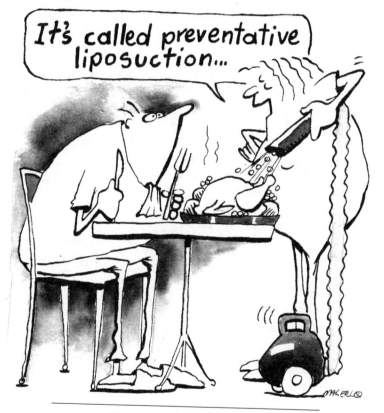

If it was possible to isolate one form of human tissue as being the most important over all others, it could conceivably be body fat. Life cannot exist without body fat. Body fat is a reservoir of essential concentrated energy without which our physical systems would fail. Body fat also envelops and protects the kidneys from physical trauma and supplies the heart with its only useable form of energy fuel. But, while a little body fat is absolutely essential, a lot is unsightly, uncomfortable and life-threatening.

What has gone wrong? Why, when we have the technology to send astronauts into space are we, as a race, suffering from such problems as being overweight and obesity? The answer is simple. We are suffering because we are consuming an imbalance of foods in alarming proportions and in opposition to the evolutionary dictates of our bodies. No surviving animal species in the wild shares the human trait of being overweight and obese, simply because wild animals instinctively consume food specific to their evolutionary development. It is difficult to imagine a member of a pride of African lions refusing to go on a hunt because he or she is on a diet.

We have progressively replaced our former complementary diet which was high in protein with some fat and little carbohydrate with a diet high in carbohydrate, with little protein and even less fat. Our systems have fallen victim to the addiction of carbohydrate, an addiction so powerful it has altered the way the body manufactures energy. Instead of deriving the majority of our body energy from highly efficient stored fat, we have forced it to function almost exclusively on the inferior energy produced from carbohydrate. The current dietary fad is to remove fat from the diet in the misguided belief that saturated fat is the sole cause of obesity, elevated serum cholesterol and serum triglycerides, cardiovascular disease and stroke. In the absence of conclusive scientific evidence, we are encouraged to eat large quantities of fruit, vegetables and grain products simply because they are cholesterol free. Yet carbohydrate foods are the single greatest contributors to the formation and retention of body fat, and indirectly to the incidence of many diseases.

If we are to understand what has gone wrong, we must first be aware of how the body reacts to various foods.

THE ROLE OF DIETARY FATS

Fats do have other roles to play in the body, but their primary function is energy production. The conversion of dietary fat into energy-ready fat is a simple process involving the absorption of triglycerides and their conversion into units of energy-ready fuel.

What are triglycerides?

Triglycerides are the major components of all the saturated and unsaturated fats and oils we consume. The triglycerides contained in saturated fats differ little from those found in unsaturated fats except unsaturated fats tend to contain more smaller or short chain triglycerides. Unsaturated fats also contain three essential fatty acids considered necessary in good nutrition.

Many of the shorter chain triglycerides can be absorbed by the body from the food we consume without assistance. Once inside the body the short chain triglycerides are transported directly to the liver where they undergo immediate conversion into energy-ready fats. These now useable units of energy are released back into the bloodstream.

The longer chain triglycerides are too large to get through the tiny holes in the wall of the intestine. To overcome the obstacle of size, the larger triglycerides are broken down into more manageable globules in the stomach before they reach the small intestine. Once inside the body, the fragmented longer chain triglycerides are reconstructed to their original form by the action of the thyroid gland. Like their shorter chain cousins, the long chain triglycerides are transported to the liver where they undergo energy-ready processing prior to their release into the bloodstream. There is no evidence to suggest the length of the triglyceride chain influences the quality of energy production other than the energy produced is proportional to the size of the triglyceride.

The triglycerides carried by the bloodstream are available to every tissue cell in the body for the manufacture of energy. However, with diets high in carbohydrate, the body chooses the easy to access glucose at the expense of the triglycerides. Triglycerides not absorbed by the tissue cells are treated as being surplus to requirements and are engorged by the fat storage cells. In former times of feast and famine, the surplus triglycerides absorbed in days of plenty were released for the production of energy when food was in short supply. Not so today. Once absorbed by the fat cells, the majority of these energy-ready triglycerides wait in vain for a second chance at producing energy.

The simplicity of the absorption and storage process of triglycerides is no doubt the reason why dietary fats are confused as being the major cause of excessive body fat formation. But, again, this is simply not the case. The body developed this uncomplicated fat absorption pathway to ensure it has ready access to its most potent energy source. It is not the fault of the triglycerides that they are not used for the production of energy as intended. The fault lies in the over-consumption of carbohydrate.

THE ROLE OF CARBOHYDRATE

The sugars we eat come from the carbohydrate foods we consume. Carbohydrate supplies the body with limited energy, but it will also form body fat if consumed to excess. However, the conversion of sugar into fat is a much more complicated process than the storing of ingested triglycerides. All ingested sugars are immediately converted into glucose, but any glucose not used in the production of energy will be converted into body fat. This is undertaken by the liver and inside the fat cells which will convert glucose into fat and place it directly into storage. Fat formed from glucose by the liver is released back into the bloodstream to join the triglycerides from ingested fats. Again, any triglycerides not used by the cells, including the triglycerides made from glucose in the liver, will be absorbed by the fat cells and stored. Therefore, the triglycerides derived from the over-consumption of sugar are exactly the same, and suffer the same fate, as do the triglycerides from fats in the diet.

THE ROLE OF PROTEIN

Protein will also form body fat if consumed to excess, but this is by far the lesser contributor. In contrast to the dietary fat and carbohydrate conversion pathways, the conversion of protein into body fat is the most complicated.

Dietary protein supplies the body with the necessary amino acids to build almost everything other than bone, including hair, nails, skin, muscles, arteries, veins and even blood cells. However, a large percentage of amino acids, called amines, consumed in excess of immediate tissue building requirements will be converted into body fat. A lesser portion of structurally different amino acids, the ketogenic group, do not form body fat. These are converted by the liver into ammonia and then into urea, purines, amines and transamines with any surplus being extracted by the kidneys and secreted in the urine.

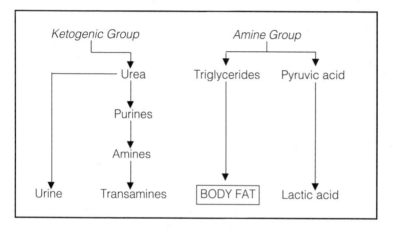

Amino Acids
Table 11.1

WHAT CAUSES EXCESS BODY FAT FORMATION?

It is apparent that all food consumed to excess is capable of forming body fat. Under ideal dietary conditions the body would receive the precise amount of carbohydrate necessary for the production of a small portion of the body's energy requirements. The body would also receive just the right amount of protein on a regular basis to supply all of the amino acids necessary for total body reconstruction. And, last but not least, the body would receive the ideal quantity of fat for the production of energy from its most potent source – triglycerides.

And the villain is . . .?

Let us now put a cat among the pigeons by increasing the daily intake of carbohydrate. Additional carbohydrate calls for additional insulin, a very active transport medium which gives glucose precedence over both triglycerides and amino acids entering the cells. The cells will usually fill to capacity with glucose, but may suffer a deficiency in the uptake of energy-ready triglycerides and amino acids. In the absence of intracellular triglycerides, the body will almost exclusively use the less potent glucose for the production of energy. It has no other choice.

Energy-ready triglycerides and amino acids denied entry into the tissue cells are forced to remain in the bloodstream. The body is left with no option other than to treat the amino acids and triglycerides as being surplus. The triglycerides are absorbed by the fat storage cells and become body fat, while the amino acids are converted into either ammonia, or into body fat.

The down side to eating carbohydrate to excess

The high carbohydrate eater is in a constant fat formation mode, a mode which effectively blocks the release of stored fat for the production of energy. Low energy glucose becomes the primary energy source with early fatigue a characteristic of daily life. Active cells are denied their quota of amino acids and triglycerides, *and the body just keeps getting fatter*.

Serum triglycerides

Although no credible link between elevated serum triglycerides and heart disease has been established, elevated serum triglycerides still attract some attention. As is the case with cholesterol, the saturated fats in our diet have been blamed for increases in the levels of blood borne triglycerides. Ironically, the preferred treatment for the condition of elevated serum triglycerides is a reduction in dietary fats and an increase in carbohydrate. But, as carbohydrate is the major contributor to the formation and retention of body fat, and to the unwanted manufacture of triglycerides, a reduction in carbohydrate intake would make more sense.

Rekindling the burning of fat

Returning to full fat burning potential is not just a matter of making changes in your diet for a day. Once the body is forced to burn glucose as its major source of energy it develops a preference for glucose over triglycerides. The fat release and triglyceride burning functions become suppressed, and this scenario takes time to reverse. The time required to complete the transformation process away from burning mostly glucose to burning mostly fat for energy will vary according to the extent and duration of your carbohydrate dependency. However, data gathered by the author suggests that majority fat burning potential can be achieved within 23 weeks, and full fat burning potential within 53 weeks of adopting a balanced eating program.

Based on your lean body weight, your *Slim Forever* program will allow you to establish your exact requirements of the essential food groups of protein, carbohydrate and fat. Your balanced intake of food will return your system to burning stored fat as its major energy source *and the fat on your body will melt away.*

The influence exerted by your change in dietary habits will not be confined to the weight loss part of your program. Your body will also be assured of an optimum intake of balanced nutrients during the weight maintenance part of your program. The only difference will be that during weight loss you will actively lose unwanted body fat, and during weight maintenance you will stabilise your chosen level of fat content. Whether you reach your desired level of weight loss prior to or after the 23 or 53-week period of balanced eating is not important. Either way you will reach your full fat burning potential within the time frame, and you will maintain it provided you follow *The golden rules of being slim forever* presented in Chapter 2.

Carbohydrate intake must remain constant

You will not have to increase your intake of carbohydrate during weight loss or weight maintenance for any reason. Even prolonged heavy work or exercise is not an exception because a body under physical load will automatically burn more fat and less glucose for energy. Therefore, the glucose you do consume will be preserved and your body will derive the additional energy it requires from high-potency triglycerides.

OPTIMUM BODY FAT LEVELS

It is important we retain a level of stored body fat, but there is some confusion as to what constitutes an optimum level of body fat.

Body fat falls into two distinct categories. The first is the inner or essential organ fat surrounding the kidneys and to a lesser degree, the heart. The second is the outer or subcutaneous layer of stored energy-ready body fat. However, the possibility of variations in distribution between internal and external body fat in individuals must be considered. Any meaningful assessment must also allow for the variation in the mass of female breast tissue, which is almost all adipose tissue.

An optimum level of body fat cannot be expressed as a specific percentage of total body weight, but rather it must be expressed as an acceptable range. For example, an acceptable range of internal body fat in both males and females would be between 2.5% and 3.5% of total body weight. An acceptable range of external body fat would be 3.5% to 7.5%, with an additional allowance of between 0.3% and 1.2% for breast tissue in the female. All factors considered, the total fat content of males should be in the range of 6% to 11%, and of females between 6.3% and 12.2% of total body weight. It must be understood that a person with a total body fat content of 7% would be just as healthy if their body fat content increased to 11%. It is the extremes of body fat content either below or above the stated ranges that cause problems.

body energy

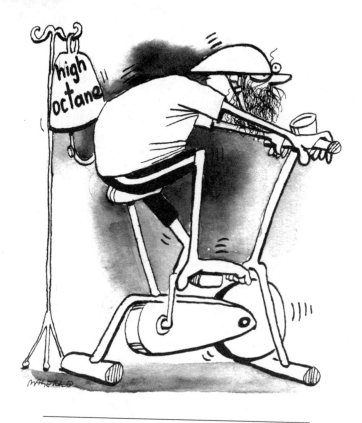

Fat not glucose is the major energy source

What influences the balance of energy production?

The litmus test of energy production

The subject of body energy is one few of us have considered other than to feel good when we have it in abundance, or wonder where it all went when we get tired.

The ergonomics of the human body can be compared with that of any energy dependent machine. Provided a flow of energy specific to a machine is constant, ongoing function is reasonably assured. But, if the energy source is interrupted, the machine, or in this case the human body, will cease to operate. Unlike simple machines capable of being restarted by putting gasoline in a tank, or by the flicking of an electrical switch, any total disruption in the supply of energy to the human body will be fatal.

The human body is capable of deriving energy from each of the major food groups. The carbohydrates and fats we consume are used almost exclusively in the production of energy, with additional energy being derived from dietary proteins consumed in excess of immediate tissue reconstruction requirements.

Precisely how the human energy system works has long been a mystery. Late in the nineteenth century scientists began seriously seeking an understanding of how the human body produces energy, and from what sources. It was apparent that both glucose and fat were involved in the production of body energy, but their precise individual and collective roles were not well defined. In the late 1960s a group of Scandinavian scientists conducted a series of tests in an effort to establish conclusively the preferential source of human energy production. The data recorded clearly supported the view that glucose was indeed the preferred and primary energy source of the human body. The evidence appeared to be conclusive, and the results were embraced by the world at large, but it is now apparent the structure of those tests was flawed.

The Scandinavian tests involved three groups of athletes fed a variety of diets over a period of six days, and then subjected to heavy exercise. The members of the first group were fed a specific diet consisting of proteins, fats and carbohydrates for the entire six day period. The members of the second group consumed a diet of only proteins and for all six days. Those in the third group were fed a diet of only proteins and fats for three days, followed by a diet consisting only of carbohydrates with no proteins or fats for the remaining three days. On the seventh day, all three groups were instructed to ride stationary indoor exercise bikes to exhaustion, and the results were recorded.

The members of the group who had been eating only proteins and fats were the first to reach exhaustion. In second place were the members of the group who had consumed a mixed diet of proteins, fats and carbohydrates. In first place were the members of the group who had consumed proteins and fats and no carbohydrates for three days, and only carbohydrates for the remaining three days. The results appeared to clearly indicate a diet consisting only of carbohydrates prior to exercise was superior to a mixed diet of proteins, fats and carbohydrates, and both were superior to a diet consisting entirely of proteins and fats. The observers concluded that carbohydrates were the major energy source of the body, and who could blame them given the evidence?

These tests were subsequently repeated on a number of occasions in other parts of the world using the same criteria, and predicably the findings in each case supported the results of the initial study. But, at no time did any of the involved scientists remotely consider the possibility that the basis of these tests was flawed, nor did they consider altering the paradigms of research in an effort to establish comparative studies.

The scientists conducting the Scandinavian inspired tests failed to consider one fact, and that was the long-term suppressive effects of carbohydrates on the availability of stored body fat for energy.

The design of the human body demands an energy mix from both fat and glucose, but what was not previously understood is the change in the balance between the two sources in response to alterations in the intensity of physical activity.

At best, the human body contains enough processed carbohy-drate in the form of free glucose, and its emergency storage form of glycogen, to last just a few hours under conditions of heavy exercise. Conversely, even a slim person has greater than 200 times more energy-ready fat available for the production of energy than is immediately available from both glucose and glycogen. Availability aside, fat is a far more potent energy source than glucose. A given quantity of fat will produce greater than $2\frac{1}{4}$ times more energy than a similar quantity of carbohydrate.

Fat in the context of energy production refers to both stored body fat and recently ingested dietary fats. Saturated and unsaturated fats supply the body with triglycerides which are made energy-ready by the liver and released into the bloodstream. The fat storage cells contain energy-ready triglycerides which are also released into the bloodstream. Therefore, any reference to fat in terms of energy production must include triglycerides from both sources.

FAT NOT GLUCOSE IS THE MAJOR ENERGY SOURCE

Current data suggests the energy mix of glucose and fat alters dramatically with any increase in physical load. It is now apparent the human body responds to heavy exercise by using more fat and less glucose in the production of energy, an assertion confirmed by tests conducted in the United States in 1986 involving competitive body builders. Selected athletes were assigned weights calculated to take them to exhaustion at the completion of 20 sets of repetitive leg exercises. Comparative pre- and post-exercise muscle testing produced some startling results. If glucose is the major source of human energy, exercising to exhaustion by these athletes would reasonably have depleted all their available stores of muscle glucose and glycogen, but it didn't. Post-exercise muscle testing indicated only 40% of the available muscle glycogen had been used, calculated as being barely enough energy to perform one set of exercises, much less 20. Where then did energy sufficient to perform the remaining 19 sets of exercises come from?

Emergency stores of liver glycogen had to be considered, but this was discounted as it had been tagged prior to the test, and no significant quantities were found in the muscles. Further examination indicated that the stores of muscle triglycerides, or fat, were significantly depleted. It was concluded that the major energy source under conditions of increased physical load is fat.

There can be little doubt the shift in emphasis between energy sources has much to do with the superior efficiency of fat in the production of energy under conditions of load, but availability of supply may also be a key factor. The human body can store only limited amounts of glucose and glycogen, but there is no apparent limit to the amount of fat a body can store. The human body will always require a combination of both glucose and fat to produce energy, but as physical load increases, so the shift in emphasis moves to burning more fat and less glucose.

The suppressive action of glucose over fat

What you eat greatly influences the production of glucose and fat for energy, as well as how your body uses those energy sources. Given a balanced diet of proteins, fats and carbohydrates, the body will store and release glucose and fat in proportion to physical demand, but any alteration in dietary balance will influence the way a body responds. A diet too high in carbohydrates will certainly produce abundant supplies of both glucose and fat, but carbohydrates consumed to excess appear to initiate a blocking action against the release of stored fat for the production of energy.

Like the active muscle cells, fat cells are unable to absorb glucose without the assistance of the hormone insulin, and provided the influence of insulin on the fat cells is not prolonged, all systems are go. However, if large quantities of excess blood glucose are present, the prolonged influence of the insulin in getting the glucose into the fat cells will effectively block the outward release of stored energy-ready triglycerides. Under balanced dietary conditions the uptake of excess glucose by the fat cells would be minimal and episodic, but in diets high in carbohydrates there is an almost constant uptake process. A little like chewing gum and whistling, the forced uptake of glucose by the fat cells, and the release of energy-ready triglycerides cannot be undertaken simultaneously. Due to the overpowering influence of the insulin, the process of energy-ready fat release is retarded, and an almost constant state of fat formation and retention is the result. The release of energy-ready triglycerides from the fat cells in response to an increase in physical activity is severely hampered. The body is now forced to rely almost entirely on glucose and glycogen for energy.

It would be reasonable to assume that once a body under physical load depletes the immediately available stores of blood glucose, the fat cells would simply respond by releasing more triglycerides, but unfortunately this is not the case. The body functions almost entirely on a demand-for-action basis, but a demand will go unheeded if the action has been suppressed for any length of time. The prolonged consumption of a diet high in carbohydrates will, in time, suppress the body's innate ability to release energy-ready fat across the entire spectrum of physical load. Any reversal of this abnormal fat retention phenomenon can only be achieved by dietary change and body re-education, and this takes time. Biochemist and physiologist Dr Greg Ellis, developer of the Somatech ultrasound body composition technology, in an interview with *Muscle and Fitness* magazine, suggests it may take 20 weeks for a body to readapt to a balanced diet higher in proteins and fats and lower in carbohydrates, and to resume the normal fat release function.

WHAT INFLUENCES THE BALANCE OF ENERGY PRODUCTION?

The shift in emphasis from burning glucose to burning fat for the production of energy under conditions of increased physical load does not happen by accident. A number of enzymes and hormones produced by the body in response to exercise exert specific control over the proportionate rate at which a body will burn fat and glucose for energy.

The enzyme citrate

Under balanced dietary conditions, citrate, a by-product of the fat burning process, is perhaps the most significant control factor over the suppression of glucose for energy. As physical load on the body increases, so too does the demand for additional energy. In the absence of citrate this demand would lead to an increase in the burning of both fat and glucose. However, citrate produced during the fat burning process actively suppresses the burning of glucose, and the body is forced to progressively use more fat. The more intense the physical load, the greater will be the production of citrate, and the more intense will be its sparing effects on available glucose.

The hormone glucagon

Glucagon also influences energy production at its source. The body concentrates some glucose into glycogen which it stores in the muscle cells and in the liver. With prolonged exercise, the supply of glucose in the cells and in the bloodstream may become exhausted. The body will respond by first converting the glycogen in the cells, and then the larger stores of glycogen in the liver, into glucose.

Produced in response to physical activity and glucose depletion, glucagon is a necessary catalyst in the transformation of glycogen stored in the liver into energy-ready glucose. But, glucagon also exerts a countering action over the hormone insulin. By suppressing the effects of insulin on blood glucose, glucagon effectively retards the rate of active uptake of glucose by the muscle cells. Paradoxically, glucagon has the dual roles of actively releasing energy-ready glucose into the bloodstream, but then exerting a limiting influence over its rate of absorption into the cells.

Again the absolute need for glucose in the energy burning process is emphasised, but so too are the sparing effects citrate and glucagon exert over glucose during heavy exercise.

Growth hormone

As its name implies, growth hormone promotes body growth in the anabolic, or construction phase, of tissue redevelopment. Growth hormone stimulates the absorption from the bloodstream of essential nutrients by the muscle cells. It also exerts a stimulating effect over the release of energy-ready triglycerides from the fat storage cells. The ongoing anabolic process of tissue reconstruction requires a constant supply of energy, which accounts for some of the energy used by the body at rest. It is of interest to note that growth hormone targets fat for the production of this energy, not glucose.

Diet plays a significant role in controlling the production of growth hormone. Protein and fat stimulate the synthesis of growth hormone, but carbohydrate suppresses it. A diet high in carbohydrate may effectively reduce bone and muscle growth, especially in the young, and suppress the active release of stored fat for essential energy production.

There can be no doubt, in terms of quantity, that the dietary intake of carbohydrate is the most critical of all food sources. Carbohydrate consumed to excess will result in the formation of unwanted body fat, the suppression of growth hormone synthesis, and the entrapment of the body's most potent source of energy, fat. Conversely, too little dietary carbohydrate will have an equally damaging effect on the body. If insufficient levels of dietary carbohydrate are consumed, the body will revert to converting essential free amino acids and active muscle tissue into glucose in a process known as gluconeogenesis. The obvious and immediate effects of muscle degradation aside, the muscle wasting effects of gluconeogenesis may lead to the potentially fatal condition of toxic ketosis.

Reassessing the scandinavian tests

If a balanced diet is the keystone to effective energy production from both glucose and fat under all conditions of physical stress — why then didn't the athletes in the first group of the Scandinavian studies who consumed a composite diet of proteins, fats and carbohydrates win the day? Given different pre-trial circumstances they would have, provided the ratio of proteins, fats and carbohydrates was in fact balanced. The Scandinavian tests simply did not take into account the time necessary for a body suffering long-term excessive carbohydrate consumption to be re-educated to burning more fat and less glucose under conditions of increased physical load.

The members of the group fed only proteins and fats would have suffered glucose depletion even before the physical endurance trials commenced. With the subsequent imposition of heavy exercise the members of this group would have soon experienced the muscle wasting effects of gluconeogenesis, and risked the possible onset of toxic ketosis.

The members of the group fed a diet of proteins, fats and carbohydrates for the entire six days would have experienced the onset of gluconeogenesis once the immediate supplies of glucose were exhausted. They too were incapable of releasing their vast supplies of stored fat for the production of energy and had to rely on limited access to glucose and glycogen.

The members of the group consuming only carbohydrates for the last three days prior to exercising appeared to deliver the best performance. These athletes dosed their systems on glucose and were able to take advantage of that extra glucose in the short-term. They too lacked the ability to release stored fat for energy, but the tests were terminated immediately they fell victim to exhaustion. The possibility of even greater energy supplies being available from stored fat was never a consideration.

Had the group fed proteins, fats and carbohydrates consumed a balanced diet over a period of at least 20 weeks, they would have significantly outperformed each of the other two groups.

This assertion is qualified by the results of laboratory tests conducted by Dr Greg Ellis. Rats fed a diet high in fat for one week performed 8% longer in endurance running trials than rats fed a diet high in carbohydrate. After another four weeks on their respective diets, the high fat diet group ran 33% longer than the rats on high carbohydrate diets.

The scientists involved in the Scandinavian tests failed to recognise the long-term suppressive effects of the over-consumption of carbohydrates on the utilisation of stored fat for the production of energy. Who could have foreseen the negative impact this simple, but understandable, miscalculation would eventually have on the people of this world?

THE LITMUS TEST OF ENERGY PRODUCTION

Nowhere is the energy deficit problem more apparent than with marathon runners. 'Hitting the wall' is an expression used by athletes to describe the sudden onset of energy depletion under conditions of extreme physical stress, a problem most of them bring on themselves. Erroneously believing glucose to be the major energy source of the human body, many athletes consume large quantities of carbohydrate on a daily basis, especially before they enter competition. But, the long-term suppressive effects of excessive carbohydrate consumption negate the athletes' natural ability to quantitatively reduce glucose utilisation and increase the demand for the release of fat energy.

The problem with carbohydrate dosing

Carbohydrate dosing prior to competition by these athletes increases their immediate supply of glucose and glycogen. But, it also drastically increases the production of insulin, and decreases the synthesis of growth hormone. After two hours or so of competitive hard running they totally exhaust their supplies of glucose and glycogen, and with little or no access to the abundance of energy contained in stored fat, they revert to breaking down essential muscle tissue. As gluconeogenesis is a process designed as a safety valve to sustain life under conditions of extreme energy depletion, it is consequently a slow and reluctant process. Gluconeogenesis produces only limited amounts of glucose, sufficient only to sustain life under resting conditions. It simply does not have the ability to supply the amount of glucose necessary to sustain heavy exercise, and it is at this point that the marathon runner hits the wall.

Conclusive evidence in support of fat for energy

The world was captivated in 1968 when Mamo Wolde, a relatively unknown Ethiopian runner, won the gold medal for the marathon at the Olympic Games in Mexico City. At the age of 36, he became the oldest athlete ever to win this prestigious event, setting a time record that stands to this day. A product of village life in Ethiopia, Wolde grew up running and hunting wild game on foot, and consuming a diet high in proteins and fats, and low in carbohydrates. Subsequent tests indicated Wolde's body, under conditions of physical load, readily switched to burning fat as its main energy source. This inspiring and talented runner was never known to hit the wall.

Athletes and non athletes alike would improve their overall physical performance, and reduce excessive stores of body fat, if they consumed a balance of the essential food groups as outlined by the *Slim Forever* program.

Author's note

My research to date in the field of energy production indicates that a person who has consumed a diet high in carbohydrate for any extended period of time will burn predominantly glucose for energy, even under conditions of heavy load. By consuming a balanced diet of proteins, fats and carbohydrates the average person will increase the burning of fat for energy to a minimum of 50% of total energy production after approximately 23 weeks. Full fat burning potential of around 90% of total body energy will not be reached before 53 weeks.

This body re-education process is further evidenced by my discovery that a body suffering the long-term effects of carbohydrate consumption will only actively reduce fat deposits for a maximum period of 5–6 hours each day without sensing starvation. Once optimum fat burning potential is reached, active fat reduction will have increased to a maximum of 18 hours each day, provided active fat loss is still sought.

The *Slim Forever* program will supply the body with a balance of glucose energy from carbohydrate, and triglyceride energy from ingested fats. As insulin production is controlled, the suppressive activity of this hormone on the release of stored fat is reduced. Growth hormone synthesis will be maximised and the body will freely release an abundance of stored fat for energy in keeping with the dictates of optimum metabolic function.

cholesterol

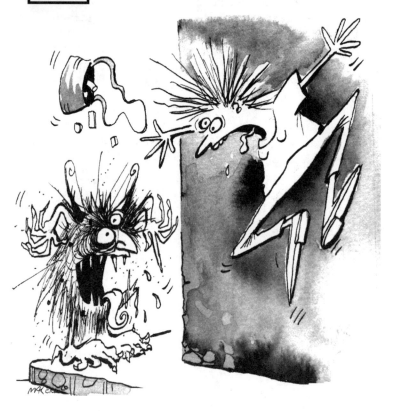

What is cholesterol

Is cholesterol both friend and foe?

What causes serum cholesterol levels to rise?

Why has cholesterol been made the scapegoat?

Arteriosclerosis

WHAT IS CHOLESTEROL?

Cholesterol is not a fat. Cholesterol is a vital fat-like substance inextricably involved in the structure, function and rebuilding of each of the estimated 75 trillion cells in the human body. This extremely important substance can be assimilated in limited amounts from the natural fats in our diet, but the majority of our requirements are supplied from internal production.

Almost every human cell is capable of synthesising cholesterol for its own use, but the liver, and to a lesser degree the small intestine, are the major sites of production. The greatest concentration of cholesterol in the human body is found in the brain. Ironically the brain is the only site known to be incapable of manufacturing cholesterol for its own use, relying entirely on cholesterol supplied from the bloodstream to fulfil its needs.

Cholesterol has many uses. The most abundant use of cholesterol, as much as 80% of all ingested and synthesised cholesterol, is in the production of cholic acid. Cholic acid is a bile salt manufactured by the liver and stored in the gall bladder. From the gall bladder it is released into the stomach where it promotes the emulsification and absorption of dietary fats. Without cholic acid most of the fats we consume would pass right on through our systems totally undigested. The existence of this intricate emulsification and absorption process, together with the ability of the body to produce cholic acid in such profusion, conclusively proves the absolute need for the inclusion of fats in our daily diet.

In addition to its indispensable role in fat absorption and tissue reconstruction, cholesterol is a key component in the manufacture of a number of hormones. Included in this list are the female sex hormones oestrogen and progesterone, and the male sex hormone testosterone. Cholesterol also binds with other fats to give skin its resistant quality to water and some chemicals, and to prevent dehydration. Without the fatty protection of cholesterol the level of surface body fluid evaporation would increase from a normal ½ pt/240 ml to a possible 5 gal/20 L each day, resulting in severe dehydration. Cholesterol in the skin also interacts with sunlight in the biosynthesis of vitamin D, an essential interactive agent with calcium in the formation of bone.

IS CHOLESTEROL BOTH FRIEND AND FOE?

Heart and blood vascular disorders are on the rise and our attention has been focused on cholesterol as the culprit. As saturated fats contain cholesterol, the inclusion of saturated fats in our diet has been blamed for the formation of excessive levels of cholesterol in the bloodstream. This rationale has gathered momentum to a point where people generally are being encouraged to reduce their intake of dietary proteins and saturated fats, and to increase their intake of unsaturated fats and carbohydrates irrespective of their relative serum cholesterol levels.

There is growing confusion and contradiction surrounding the results and interpretation of many studies involving serum cholesterol levels. Despite the current thrust aimed at reducing dietary cholesterol intake, the majority of clinical studies indicate neither increasing nor decreasing the intake of dietary saturated fats will have any appreciable effect on serum cholesterol levels. Doctor Arthur C. Guyton of the University of Mississippi School of Medicine suggests the long-term effects of raising or lowering the dietary intake of fats and cholesterol in the human will not alter serum cholesterol levels either way by greater than 15%. This is a far cry from the 300% to 400% increases currently being reported in some cases. This position is supported by Dr Robert S. Goodhart of the New York Academy of Medicine and Dr Maurice E. Shils from Cornell University Medical College who jointly assert the human body cannot absorb greater than 40% of its circulating cholesterol requirements from the diet, irrespective of the level of cholesterol in foods consumed.

Clinical tests conducted in England over a six year period clearly indicated the administration of low fat diets to heart sufferers did nothing to improve the prognosis of those patients. In reviewing this and a number of similar experiments, Dr Goodhart and Dr Shils reached the conclusion that tests involving humans have not conclusively proven lowering dietary cholesterol in any way prevented or reduced the incidence of heart disease or coronary mortality.

Yet further evidence is offered by Dr Helen Andrews Guthrie, Professor of Nutrition at Pennsylvania State University, who comments that tests involving the restriction of cholesterol-containing foods such as eggs, meat and liver led neither to a lowering of blood cholesterol levels, nor to a reduction in heart disease in humans.

The release in December 1991 of the results of a 15-year study conducted in Finland sent shock waves through the scientific and medical communities. Six hundred and twelve overweight business executives considered at risk of heart disease were persuaded to join a control group. They were encouraged to reduce or eliminate smoking and the consumption of alcohol, undertake fat lowering dietary changes and exercise regularly. A like number of high risk executives were encouraged to continue with their current lifestyle and change nothing. Records kept over a period of 15 years clearly indicate the incidence of heart attacks and deaths attributable to heart disease were $2\frac{1}{2}$ times higher among those in the control group than those in the non-control group.

A review of the many diet and lifestyle alteration studies conducted worldwide indicates that although heart attacks and cardiac deaths may be reduced among some patients on low fat diets, the overall death rate either remains the same, or increases. At best there has been a shift in the cause of death suggesting either that fat in the diet is not the villain, or, if the disease does not get you the cure surely will.

Eliminating fat from the diet is obviously not the answer. Ann Louise Gittleman, the former Director of Nutrition at the Pritikin Center in Santa Monica, California, reports some long-term participants of the Pritikin no fat diet program subsequently presented with uncontrollable weight gain, insatiable hunger and nutritional deficiencies. These conditions she relates to the absence of fat in their recommended diets. Where Pritikin saw fat as the problem, Gittleman was seeing it as the solution, describing fat as 'one of the most basic yet least understood nutrients'.

If we were to accept the hype surrounding serum cholesterol levels we could be forgiven for believing elevated serum cholesterol is a problem confronting us all. But this is not the case. Perhaps only one in every four people have detectible serum cholesterol readings above the levels considered acceptable by the World Health Organization, yet we are all urged to change our dietary habits. As the major cause of death among the 75% of the population who register normal serum cholesterol levels is heart disease, the validity of the serum cholesterol theory and the low fat high carbohydrate diet regimen must be challenged.

Are unsaturated fats the answer?

Our quest for lower serum cholesterol levels has given rise to our current obsession of replacing saturated fats with unsaturated oils, but again evidence in support of such recommendations is not conclusive. Data now suggests our focus should be directed at the type rather than the quantity of fats we consume. Eskimos in their natural habitat consume a diet averaging 70% fat, some protein and very little carbohydrate, yet heart disease is almost unknown to these people. Gittleman suggests the answer to this apparent paradox may lie in the high concentrations of the omega-3 group of fatty acids found in the cold water fish that constitute a large part of the Eskimos' diet.

Doctor Ross Hume Hall the Professor of Biochemistry at McMaster University in Canada compares the dietary fat intake of people living in northern and southern India. People in the north consume large quantities of saturated butter fat with 98% of their fat intake classified as being saturated. Yet the incidence of cardiovascular disease is exceptionally low in this area. By comparison, people living in the south consume little total fat, but 45% of the fat they do consume is classified as being polyunsaturated. Yet these people display an incidence of cardiovascular disease seven times higher than their northern cousins.

Evidence offered by Dr Goodhart and Dr Shils raises yet another question regarding the balance of fats in our diet. They assert the absorption rate of dietary cholesterol into the body is greater in the presence of unsaturated oils than with saturated fats. This being the case, the inclusion of unsaturated vegetable oils in the diet may facilitate rather than hinder dietary cholesterol uptake.

On the other hand, mono-unsaturated oils appear to exert some positive influence over already elevated serum cholesterol levels. Independent studies conducted in the United States suggest mono-unsaturated oils such as olive and peanut oils do more to prevent the formation of arterial clogging plaque than do low fat high carbohydrate diets.

The consumption of saturated fats has been shown to reduce serum cholesterol levels as evidenced by the results of a recent United States study involving sufferers of elevated serum cholesterol. In an interview with *Muscle & Fitness* magazine, biochemist and physiologist Dr Greg Ellis stated that members of a control group were placed on a diet of rib eye steaks with limited carbohydrate. The serum cholesterol levels of the people participating in the experiment significantly decreased from an average of 263 mg per 100 ml/7.1 millimoles per L to 189 mg per 100 ml/5.1 millimoles per L as compared to a recommended maximum level at that time of 205 mg per 100 ml/5.5 millimoles per L.

WHAT CAUSES SERUM CHOLESTEROL LEVELS TO RISE?

The volume of available evidence suggests the real problem may not be the cholesterol we eat or produce, but rather the cholesterol we accumulate in our bloodstream. This being the case, the question of possible overproduction of cholesterol must be tempered with the question of possible under-utilisation. Any attempt at qualifying the causes of elevated serum cholesterol must embrace an understanding of the interrelationship between diet and associated bodily function.

To appreciate the complexities of serum cholesterol accumulation, an unbiased study must consider the importance of the roles played in the production process by:

1 cholic acid;

2 acetyl CoA;

3 the phospholipid lecithin; and

4 the lipoproteins.

The role of cholic acid

The body uses approximately 80% of all available cholesterol in the manufacture of cholic acid. Synthesised by the liver in response to the amount of fats consumed in the diet, the bile salt cholic acid is stored in the gall bladder and released into the stomach on demand. Like the action of dishwashing liquid on fats and oils in the kitchen sink, cholic acid dissolves dietary fats to render them soluble in water and readily absorbable by the intestine.

The initial site of internal cholesterol synthesis is within the wall of the small intestine. Production is controlled by the detected presence or absence of cholic acid in the food being absorbed. But, as the amount of cholic acid released from the gall bladder is proportional to the amount of fats present in the stomach, the greater the volume of fats consumed, the greater will be the volume of cholic acid released.

However, the control cholic acid places on the production of intestinal cholesterol is inversely proportional to its level of concentration in the food being absorbed. That is to say, if the concentration of fats is high, so too will be the concentration of cholic acid, which in turn will signal the intestine not to produce cholesterol as there is plenty on the way. Conversely, if the concentration of fats in the stomach is low the amount of cholic acid released will also be low, and the intestine will respond by increasing cholesterol production. This inherent mechanism ensures the low fat dieter is beaten even before the nutrients he or she consumes ever reach the bloodstream.

To summarise, diets high in fats will initiate an increased demand for cholic acid synthesis by the liver, while diets low in fats will cause a decrease in production. Any decrease in the manufacture of cholic acid leads to an under-utilisation of liver cholesterol. As unused liver cholesterol is dumped into the bloodstream, low cholic acid production may in turn give rise to an increase in serum cholesterol levels.

Therefore:

$\downarrow$ **dietary fats** = $\downarrow$ **cholic acid** = $\uparrow$ **serum cholesterol**

The role of acetyl CoA

Both the liver and the small intestine rely entirely on a non-dietary substance called acetyl CoA for the production of cholesterol. As acetyl CoA is produced in the liver during the conversion of triglycerides into energy, saturated fats have been blamed for increases in acetyl CoA levels. However, acetyl CoA is also produced during the conversion of unsaturated triglycerides into energy, and in the synthesis of triglycerides from excess blood glucose.

Doctor James M. Orten, Professor of Biochemistry at Wayne University, and Dr Otto W. Neuhaus, Professor of Biochemistry at the University of South Dakota, confirm the action of carbohydrates on the production of acetyl CoA by the liver. They claim diets high in carbohydrate give rise to an increase in the production of triglycerides from glucose, and a corresponding increase in the available pool of acetyl CoA. Therefore, the internal production of cholesterol associated with low fat high carbohydrate diets may well be attributable to the over-consumption of fruit, vegetables and sugar laden foods, not fat. They also assert that the only known control factor over the internal synthesis of triglycerides from glucose by the liver is dietary fat. Carbohydrates stimulate the production of acetyl CoA in the liver, but dietary fats act in reverse by suppressing the production of the enzyme acetyl CoA carboxylase and the citrate lyase, necessary ingredients in the internal production of triglycerides.

Therefore, any increase in the dietary intake of carbohydrate accompanied by a decrease in the intake of dietary fat will result in an increase in the production of acetyl CoA in the liver, and probably serum cholesterol.

Therefore:

$\uparrow$ **carbohydrate** = $\uparrow$ **acetyl CoA** = $\uparrow$ **serum cholesterol**

The role of the phospholipid lecithin

Lecithin is an essential fatty phospholipid produced in almost every cell in the body. Like cholesterol, it is synthesised primarily in the liver and in the wall of the small intestine from the fats we eat. Lecithin is also a member of the bile salt family, working in conjunction with cholic acid to dissolve fats in the stomach in preparation for absorption into the body. The function of lecithin in emulsifying serum cholesterol is similar to its role as a bile salt. Doctor Orten and Dr Neuhaus describe phospholipids as 'biologic detergents'. The emulsifying effect of lecithin on blood borne triglycerides and cholesterol renders these substances more easily absorbable by the tissue cells.

Molecules of cholesterol in the bloodstream tend to clump together, making them too large to gain access through the tiny holes in the cell walls. This clumping action may also contribute to the tendency of serum cholesterol to stick to the sides of the arteries. The role of lecithin is to separate and emulsify the clumps of cholesterol and reduce them to a size acceptable to absorption by the cells.

Significant reductions in serum cholesterol levels in some patients have been recorded following the administration of oral lecithin. Egg whites are an excellent source of lecithin, a point apparently overlooked by those who champion a restriction in the number of eggs we consume.

Lecithin has a fully active life of little more than 24 hours once it reaches the bloodstream. Even the occasional consumption of fats will not be sufficient to stimulate the production of lecithin in quantities necessary for the emulsification of serum cholesterol. Large clumps of cholesterol not subjected to the emulsifying action of lecithin are denied entry into the cells, and serum cholesterol levels will rise.

Therefore:

$$\downarrow \text{ dietary fats} = \downarrow \text{ lecithin} = \uparrow \text{ serum cholesterol}$$

The role of high density lipoproteins

High density lipoproteins (HDL) are a triad of nutrients manufactured by the body from approximately:

1 50% protein;

2 30% fat in the form of phospholipid; and

3 20% cholesterol.

HDL and lecithin work as a team. HDL act as carriers which seek out and attach themselves to the molecules of emulsified cholesterol and actively transport them back to the cells. Without HDL as vehicles, the cargo cholesterol would remain in the bloodstream.

Any reduction in the concentration of HDL will lead to a reduction in the amount of serum cholesterol absorbed by the cells and an increase in serum cholesterol levels. As HDL are made from protein, fat and cholesterol, any reduction in the dietary intake of these nutrients must impinge upon their production.

Therefore:

$$\downarrow \text{ dietary fats} = \downarrow \text{ HDL} = \uparrow \text{ serum cholesterol}$$

Low fat high carbohydrate dietary modifications are threatening our very existence. If we again consume a balance of nutrients in accordance with the laws of our four million years of development we could eliminate the problems caused by being overweight or obese, and the many associated diseases *forever.*

Are there two types of cholesterol?

There is a widely held misconception that there are two types of cholesterol. The high density lipoproteins (HDL) have been labelled by some researchers as good cholesterol while the low density lipoproteins (LDL) have been isolated as being bad cholesterol. However lipoproteins, be they of high or low density, are not cholesterol.

There are in fact four members of the lipoprotein family. In addition to HDL and LDL the body also manufactures very low density lipoproteins (VLDL) and chylomicrons. These various lipoproteins are classified according to the concentrations of protein, fat and cholesterol of which they are formed, and their function.

All four categories of lipoproteins are found in the blood stream. The chylomicrons transport ingested fats from the intestine to the tissue cells, while the VLDL carry the triglycerides manufactured by the liver from glucose to the tissue cells. The role of the LDL has not yet been established, however, one theory suggests that LDL may be the first step in the natural destruction of VLDL once their role in the transportation of triglycerides from the liver is completed. As previously stated, the HDL are the medium used in the transport of cholesterol from the bloodstream and into the tissue cells.

It would appear that the confusion between lipoproteins and cholesterol may be rooted in the knowledge that high ratios of HDL over LDL usually accompany low serum cholesterol levels, while a predominance of LDL is usually found in association with high serum cholesterol levels. A diet high in carbohydrate will cause an increase in the production of triglycerides by the liver from excess glucose and initiate a corresponding increase in the production of VLDL. This will in turn lead to an increase in the level of serum LDL. A diet low in fat will inhibit the necessary production of HDL which will in turn suppress the absorption of serum cholesterol by the tissue cells. Therefore, a low HDL and high LDL serum count is probably the result of eating too much carbohydrate and too little fat, and not too much saturated fat as has been suggested.

WHY HAS CHOLESTEROL BEEN MADE THE SCAPEGOAT?

The presence of cholesterol in arterial plaque cannot be denied, but cholesterol is just one of a number of ingredients necessary for the formation of plaque.

Doctor Wally Cliff of the Cardiovascular Pathology Unit at the Australian National University argues that cholesterol has been overemphasised. He believes our current obsession with diet and lifestyle may have blinded medical science to other possible explanations for heart disease. The post-mortem examination of approximately 200 human hearts by Dr Cliff and his colleague Dr Gutta Shoefl isolated a fibrous build-up of collagen, the substance ligaments and tendons are made of, in the coronary artery of cardiac suffers. Doctor Cliff suggests the inflammation and collagen formation associated with coronary disease may be the body's immune system responding to toxic, viral or bacterial infection, and any cholesterol build-up may be incidental (Julian Cribb, 'The great debate about cholesterol', *The Weekend Australian,* 21 March 1992).

Cholesterol has been made the scapegoat due to persistent misinterpretation of the presenting facts. Arterial plaque is currently considered a precursor to a large proportion of diagnosed cardiac disease sufferers. And, as arterial plaque contains cholesterol, cardiac disease has been linked to increases in serum cholesterol levels. Saturated fats came under fire simply because saturated fats are the only food source known to contain cholesterol. Immediate dietary recommendations were made encouraging everyone to restrict their intake of saturated fats; to increase the consumption of unsaturated fats; and to increase the consumption of foods of the carbohydrate group.

This rationalisation of a complex issue without the benefit of all of the facts has served to exacerbate rather than diminish the original problem. Instead of having just a rise in cardiac disease we now have an unprecedented rise in the conditions of being overweight and obesity, and their many associated diseases, including cardiac disease. Cholesterol has been branded the villain in heart disease, but there is a developing ground swell of information clearly suggesting that cholesterol has been wrongly accused.

ARTERIOSCLEROSIS

Almost half of all human deaths are attributable to the accumulation of plaque associated with arteriosclerosis, two-thirds of those from heart disease.

What is arteriosclerosis?

Arteriosclerosis literally means 'hardening of the arteries', but by common usage it has come to include any condition involving thickening and loss of elasticity of the wall of an artery. In the case of heart disease the arteries most commonly affected are those in immediate proximity to the heart itself.

Loss of elasticity of an artery reduces the magnitude of the pulsations of the affected artery which would otherwise assist the heart in propelling blood around the body. Arterial wall thickening due to deposits of fatty plaque occludes the inside or lumen of an artery, reducing the volume of blood it can carry. In an attempt to overcome these obstacles and keep the blood flowing, the heart must pump harder and faster. This increased load on the heart may ultimately cause it to fail in what we call a heart attack. Increases in both the rate of contraction and the pressure of contraction exert a strain on the arteries themselves, and this pressure may cause them to burst. The rupture of a blood vessel to the brain placed under such pressure is the cause of most strokes.

What causes arterial plaque?

Plaque formation is usually associated with degenerative changes in the arterial wall itself, damage that may well be attributed, at least in part, to the effects of ingested toxic substances. Evidence now suggests food additives, damaged oils and fats, the prolonged use of some medication and the excessive consumption of coffee may all be contributing factors in the formation of arterial plaque.

Blood borne toxins are believed to attack and damage the cells of the normally smooth and slippery interior surface of the arteries. As a result, rough patches form on the surface of the artery which in turn impede the free flow of blood borne fats and cholesterol. Doctor Guyton suggests arterial wall damage caused by the persistent pressure of hypertension may precipitate the formation of plaque. Irrespective of the cause, arterial wall damage appears to be an accepted precursor to the formation of arterial plaque.

Some researchers have attempted to solve the problem of arterial plaque formation by conducting experiments involving animals. For example, arterial plaque can be easily produced in rabbits by feeding them cholesterol, but these animals are natural vegetarians. Being herbivores, rabbits appear to lack the humanly inherent ability to reduce the internal production of cholesterol in response to increased dietary intake. This being the case, the introduction of cholesterol, a substance not normally found in the rabbits' diet, must initiate a gross accumulation of serum cholesterol. It simply has nowhere else to go.

The production of arterial plaque in meat eating animals has also been achieved, but this presented as a much more difficult task. Induced arterial plaque has been recorded in dogs following the removal of the animal's thyroid gland, and the post-operative administration of diets excessively high in cholesterol. Such findings must be discounted out of hand as the method of producing the result is bizarre in the extreme. Unfortunately, data such as this is often presented in argument as proof positive of the effects of increased dietary cholesterol on serum cholesterol levels without due emphasis being given to the methodology employed in gathering such information.

Who is at risk of arteriosclerosis?

Arterial plaque is primarily a disease of the aged, but time rather than the age of the person is the key. Arterial plaque does not occur overnight. It is the culmination of a lifetime of fat deposition arising from a variety of influencing factors. Doctor Stanley L. Robbins of the Boston University School of Medicine verifies that fatty streaking of the coronary artery is detectible in every person by age 15 years. In some cases these fatty streaks increase in both number and severity over many years, often progressing to arteriosclerosis. Why fatty streaking disappears in some individuals and increases in others is unknown.

The incidence of arterial plaque formation is most common in men, especially between the ages of 45 and 54 years. Pre-menopausal women are affected less than men of similar age, but post-menopausal women are affected almost equally as men of the same age group. This delayed change in the disposition of women to arterial plaque formation is believed to be associated with the loss of the probable protective effects of the sex hormone oestrogen. Work related stress is also considered a factor affecting men, but with the emergence of greater female influence in the work place, the disparity between men and women affected by stress related heart disorders may diminish.

Elevated serum cholesterol levels appear to be contributing risk factors in the formation of arterial plaque, but so too are obesity, hypertension, cigarette smoking and ailments such as hypercholesterolemia, diabetes mellitus, hypothyroidism and kidney disease. The Framington study involving 2000 men between the ages of 30 and 59 years, indicated the recorded incidence in deaths from heart disease increased significantly when multiple risk factors were present. Using men with no risk factors as a basis for comparison, the mortality rate from heart disease among men with one risk factor doubled. Men with two detectible risk factors recorded a fourfold increase in cardiac mortality, while those exhibiting three risk factors had a death rate from heart disease seven times higher than members of the no risk group.

Although significant, the above study did not take into account the relative physical activity of the members of the study group. In a study concentrating on the physical activity levels of the participants, it was discovered that those who were the least physically active had a death rate from heart disease three times greater than those who were the most physically active (Robbins, Stanley L., *Pathologic Basis of Disease,* 1974).

Our forebears had to run their food down, but we need do nothing more physically taxing than driving to the local supermarket. Or, we may even have our food home delivered. Regular cardiovascular exercise is an important ingredient in achieving and maintaining an acceptable level of health and well-being, and a life relatively free of heart disease. If the prediction suggesting a 75% decrease in the incidence of all disease could be achieved with regular daily exercise is correct, then lack of exercise may well be our number one cause of death.

Hereditary and acquired diseases contribute to both elevations in serum cholesterol levels and to the onset of arteriosclerosis. With the condition known as inherited hypercholesterolemia, serum cholesterol levels continue to rise irrespective of the person's diet. Many sufferers of hereditary atherosclerosis experience the formation of arterial plaque despite serum cholesterol levels often found to be within the accepted normal range. The severe onset of either diabetes mellitus (often associated with excessive sugar intake) or hypothyroidism will frequently precede the development of premature and severe arterial plaque. Similarly, sufferers of hypertension display a level of heart disease associated with arteriosclerosis twice that of people with normal blood pressure readings.

The French paradox

What has become known as the French paradox is the confussion arising from the apparent conflict in understanding why the people of France, who consume more butter, cream and saturated fat than any other western population, display one of the lowest incidence of heart disease in the world.

Evidence derived from controlled tests conducted around the world suggest the reason for the low incidence of heart disease in France is directly related to the inclusion of fresh saturated fats in the diet and not in spite of it.

What is the answer?

The answer to the high incidence of heart disease and plaque related diseases may well be found in:

- modifying the intake of carbohydrates;

- including fish protein in the diet;

- consuming a balance of essential fats;

- reducing the intake of food chemicals and coffee;

- modifying the unnecessary scripting of medication;

- moderating the consumption of alcohol;

- not smoking; and

- undertaking moderate daily exercise.

'What's left?' you ask. Nothing really, other than good health, a wonderful feeling of physical and mental well-being, and the promise of a long and vibrant life.

Nothing in this chapter should be construed as suggesting the indiscriminate consumption of fats will not be deleterious to your health. Saturated and unsaturated fats form an essential part of our daily diet, but balance and moderation in accordance with the *Slim Forever* philosophy is the key to good health.

What level of serum cholesterol is desirable?

There is always difficulty in establishing a *normal* range for any body function, and serum cholesterol is no exception. No stated range is absolute as some individuals may register within a suggested range but in fact be deficient or excessive, while others may register outside the range and be totally normal. In establishing a normal range for any function, a representative group of people are assessed and the range occupied by the greater number of participants is deemed to be the acceptable normal range. Individuals with readings higher or lower than the majority are automatically categorised as being abnormal.

The acceptable upper limit of serum cholesterol as determined by the World Health Organization (WHO) was 205 mg per 100 ml/5.5 millimoles per L. More recent suggestions place this figure at 180 mg per 100 ml/4.85 millimoles per L. In the light of available evidence it would be interesting to know what paradigms are used by WHO in establishing these suggested levels. Data suggests elevated serum cholesterol alone constitutes no greater threat, and in some cases less threat, than other factors associated with heart disease. In the absence of long-term studies involving groups of people with blood cholesterol readings at all levels, both alone and in association with combinations of other risk factors, any suggested desirable level of serum cholesterol must be presumed arbitrary.

Also of concern is that all studies involving serum cholesterol have included only males. It is becoming evident that females may have naturally higher serum cholesterol levels than do males, perhaps as much as 25 mg per 100 ml/0.7 millimoles per L. This being the case, some females may be attempting to achieve serum cholesterol levels which are too low.

Notwithstanding, good health dictates all body functions, including serum cholesterol levels, should be maintained within reasonable bounds. If your serum cholesterol levels are elevated and you do not suffer from any of the organic or genetically acquired diseases previously mentioned, the short-term taking of oral lecithin is usually very effective. This naturally safe and essential compound is inexpensive and is readily available from most health stores and pharmacies. Long-term reductions of serum cholesterol levels can be achieved by consuming a balanced diet of proteins, fats and carbohydrates as outlined in the *Slim Forever* program.

The inevitable exception

There is one exception to the serum cholesterol rule. If you engage in heavy exercise, especially weight lifting or body building, your serum cholesterol level will increase quite naturally in response to a demand for increased tissue reconstruction. With the imposition of heavy exercise your serum cholesterol level will rise by as much as 40%, but this will be normal for you under these conditions. A sustained increase in serum cholesterol in association with heavy exercise is not only absolutely safe, it is necessary if optimum metabolic function is to be achieved and maintained. With the cessation of heavy exercise your serum cholesterol will return to its previous level, usually within 21 days.

1⁄4 *steak and eggs*

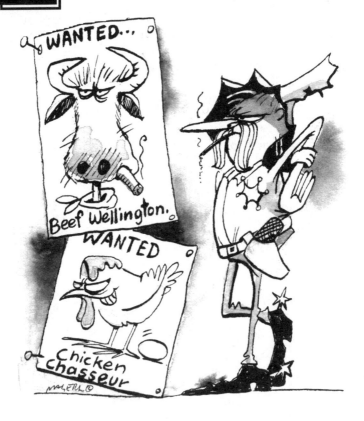

In defence of red meat

The much maligned egg

IN DEFENCE OF RED MEAT

Red meat, like poultry and fish, is a complete protein source. That is to say, red meat contains all 19 essential and non essential amino acids and is therefore capable of providing the human body with all of the necessary ingredients for muscle and tissue development and maintenance.

Our bodies do not differentiate between food sources in selecting nutrients. In the case of protein, a molecule of any amino acid from a vegetable, or from a piece of chicken or fish, is the same as a molecule of that same amino acid from red meat. The colour of the meat matters little, other than the concentration of some individual amino acids may be greater in one source than in another.

Exploding the myths

The validity of red meat as a food source has been seriously undermined over recent years. The eating of red meat has been cited as the cause of aggressive behavioural patterns; increases in serum cholesterol levels; hypertension; heart attacks; and a variety of digestive and pregnancy disorders. These claims have since been abandoned by the scientific community.

The former belief that the consumption of large amounts of red meat may damage the kidneys or liver has never been supported by scientific observation. More recent studies show diets containing ample amounts of protein very often improve the healing tendency in liver and kidney diseases. In fact, it has been conclusively established that people with diets consisting predominantly of meat do not develop any pathological symptoms, even after many years (Goodhart, R.S. and Shils, M.E., *Modern Nutrition in Health and Disease – Dietotherapy,* 1976).

The association of aggressive human behaviour with the eating of too much red meat cannot be substantiated. Some meat eating animals may appear more aggressive than do their herbivorous counterparts, but the carnivores' innate tendency to kill is based on a need to eat to survive, an act performed without malice, and devoid of wilful aggression. Apart from satisfying a need for food, meat eating animals rarely attack or fight unless they are provoked, unlike the water buffalo which is perhaps the most unpredictable and aggressive of all animals, and it is herbivorous.

Is red meat difficult to digest?

The digestive rate of red meat has been grossly misinterpreted. The assertion that red meat eaters have pounds of partially digested chunks of red meat stuck in their intestine is absurd. The digestion of all food commences in the mouth where the process of chewing, provided it is undertaken correctly, reduces the food to a pulp before it is swallowed. Upon entering the stomach the food undergoes further and more concentrated digestion by the addition of enzymes and hydrochloric acid. When the food reaches an acceptable level of digestion, it is released into the intestine where the absorption of nutrients into the bloodstream takes place. Red meat, like all other food substances, is not released from the digestive process of the stomach until it has achieved an acceptable level of preabsorption consistency.

Red meat may take a little longer than vegetable and other meat sources to complete the digestion process, but this extension of time is registered in hours, not days. The connective tissue in red muscle meat is stronger than the connective tissue found in red organ meat, poultry and fish, and takes longer to predigest. It is the breaking down of the connective tissue found in the meat itself that differentiates one protein source from another in terms of digestive time.

Far from being harmful, the additional time taken in breaking down the connective tissue of red muscle meat may actually be beneficial. The nutrient content of any food entering the small intestine en masse is not as well absorbed as when food is released in lesser amounts. The slower digestive rate of red muscle meat and the subsequent slower rate of release into the intestine may contribute to more efficient nutrient absorption. Further, proteins and fats are appetite suppressors, as opposed to carbohydrates which are appetite stimulants. The delayed time release of red meat into the digestive system satiates the appetite over a longer period, and reduces the perceived need to eat.

Is eating meat and vegetables together harmful?

Also in contention are claims suggesting certain foods, especially steak and potato, should not be consumed together due to a difference in their relative acid or alkaline levels. Not so. The entire digestive process in the stomach is acid, and food leaving the stomach undergoes an acid neutralising process before it enters the intestine. This is done in the duodenum, the next port of call after the stomach, which secretes an alkaline substance in response to the perceived level of residual hydrochloric acid in the food. Therefore, all food, irrespective of its predigested natural acid or alkaline level, undergoes acidic digestion, followed by alkaline induced neutralisation.

The major role of the digestion process is to reduce all foods consumed to the smallest possible particles. This is achieved first by chewing, and then the addition of enzymes and hydrochloric acid in the stomach. As the food is reduced to a digestible consistency, called chyme, it is sent on its way. The foods with the least resistance to the action of the digestive fluids are the first to leave the stomach. These are followed in turn by foods according to their increasing resistance to digestibility, with red muscle meat bringing up the rear. If necessary, the stomach will increase production of the digestive fluids to meet the demands of the more acid resistant foods. However, if a person continues to snack on less resistant carbohydrate foods, the acid level in the stomach will remain relatively low. Although red muscle meat will digest at lower levels of acidity, it will take longer. Therefore, the delay in the digestion of red meat in some cases may be more the product of eating too much carbohydrate than of eating red meat.

Any increase in the concentration of enzymes and hydrochloric acid in the stomach is well within the capabilities of the stomach, and as all foods are neutralised in the duodenum. Red muscle meat entering the intestine is as acid neutral as any other digested food, including potato.

Is red meat acid forming?

We tend to think of food as being acid or alkaline when it is still in its predigested form, and often believe we should eat a balance of foods complementary to the maintenance of the acid balance within our bodies. The macrobiotic diets of the 1950s and 60s made famous by the San Francisco 'flower people' were developed around the Chinese Yin and Yang philosophy of balancing the acidity and alkalinity of foods. Based on the staple of brown rice, these diets proved to be nutritionally inadequate. Many young people suffered the bone deforming disease of rickets, and showed signs of the protein deficiency disease kwashiorkor. What we believe to be true about the acidity or alkalinity of the various foods we consume may in fact be the opposite to what happens when these foods enter the body.

Red and white meat, including seafood, and grains such as barley, rye, corn, wheat and wheat flour, and plums are all acid forming foods. From these foods we gain essential sulphuric, phosphoric and uric acids. The body controls the internal level of these acids by neutralising the excesses and discharging the residue in the urine.

The common varieties of fruit and vegetables, including citrus fruit which are acid in their predigested state, have an alkaline effect on the body. The citric, tartaric and lactic acids these foods contain are immediately neutralised by the body into carbon dioxide and water. The carbon dioxide is discharged through the lungs on exhalation and the water is excreted as urine.

Dairy products, some vegetable oils, onions and sugar are neutral foods and form neither acids nor alkalies.

Our bodies have developed a proven and efficient mechanism for monitoring and correcting the acid balance of the food we consume, a balance which appears not to need any external help.

Apart from its high biological value as a complete protein food, red meat, and especially liver, is an excellent source of body-ready iron. Iron is a necessary ingredient in the formation of haemoglobin in the blood, the vehicle used to transport oxygen from the lungs to every cell in the body. Red meat also contains respectable quantities of calcium, vitamins A, B_1, B_2, E and niacin, nutrients essential in maintaining balanced human biological function.

Cholesterol in red meat

The single greatest contributor to the defamation of red meat as a viable food source has been the cholesterol scare. The attempt to link ingested saturated fats with increased serum cholesterol levels focused squarely on red meat as the major culprit. A prominent factor overlooked is that most red meat contains 50% saturated fat and 50% unsaturated fat, and not 100% saturated fat as the public have been led to believe. As most red meat is consumed fresh, the fat it contains is fresh and essentially nourishing to the human body, provided it is not eaten to excess. Fresh fats have been named the culprits in arteriosclerosis, but they may not contribute to the problem of arterial plaque at all. Emerging evidence suggests it is the rancid or heat damaged fats and oils, such as those found in hydrogenated commercial cooking oils and margarine, that do the damage (Gittleman, A.L., *Beyond Pritikin*, 1989).

The processing of red meat into various forms of cold sausage such as salami and frankfurters must be questioned, as must the preparation of some fast foods. Fats quickly spoil and become rancid when exposed to air. This oxidation process renders otherwise healthy fats toxic to the human body. Oxidised fats and oils disrupt and block the normal utilisation of essential undamaged fats by the body and are known to damage artery walls, an apparent necessary precursor to atherosclerotic plaque formation.

History and the consumption of red meat

The human race evolved eating red meat. The discovery by Robert Dart in 1924 of the fossilised remains of *Australopithecus africanus*, a species of early man, served to confirm two important historical facts regarding our dietary past. Firstly, the discovery was made near the Kalahari Desert in southern Africa, an area so arid there could not have been sufficient food available to support a fruit eating vegetarian. Secondly, the cave in which this fossilised early human was discovered was strewn with bones, not that of birds or fish, but of devoured red meat animals.

The eating of red meat is deeply rooted in our early development. Robert Ardrey, in his excellent book *African Genesis,* addresses our meat eating past by examining the tooth structure of the early human. He suggests human teeth are too small and thinly enamelled with crowns 'totally inadequate for the endless grinding and munching of a vegetarian creature who must gain from low calorie foodstuffs daily nourishment to support a fair sized body'. Our eye or canine teeth, so named because they are the remnants of fang-like appendages similar to those of the meat eating dog, add further testimony to the debate. These sharp, heavily rooted teeth were designed for the ripping and tearing of meat, not the nibbling of leaves and nuts.

Red meat, along with a little fresh fat, is a nourishing and essential food source, as are the other protein sources of poultry, fish and dairy products. There is no rule of thumb to suggest how much of each source we should consume, or that any one protein source is superior to another. All meats, irrespective of their colour, are capable of supplying the human body with total protein.

Steak lovers take heart. You can live a long and very healthy life eating just red or just white meat, but as variety is the spice of life, a selection from each of the food groups is probably the most satisfying.

THE MUCH MALIGNED EGG

It is incredible to think something as nutritionally complete as the innocuous hen's egg could earn the adverse reputation it has over the past few years. The simple hen's egg contains every single vitamin, mineral, protein and fat necessary to create a total living organism. Yet, it has been blamed for conditions ranging from hives to elevated serum cholesterol, all without a modicum of evidence or truth.

This biologically complete food source contains all 19 amino acids of the protein group, saturated and unsaturated fats, calcium, iron, folic acid, niacin and vitamins A, B_1, B_2, B_3, B_6 and B_{12}. Yet nature, in its wisdom, did not add carbohydrate to this highly nutritious cocoon of life.

Much of the furore over eating eggs is again a direct result of the cholesterol scare. The cholesterol in an egg is contained in the yolk, the part of the egg that actually forms the chicken in a fertilised egg. The presence of cholesterol in the yolk serves to reinforce the absolute need for this substance in the body building and life processes. But, the cholesterol content of the egg is only half of the story. The white of the egg is rich in lecithin, the phospholipid essential for the emulsification of cholesterol in the blood prior to absorption by the individual cells of the body. The egg not only supplies essential cholesterol, but it also supplies the lecithin necessary to make it biologically complementary. In the case of the egg, the balance of lecithin to cholesterol is apparently that deemed necessary by nature to initiate optimum cellular uptake and tissue growth.

Any suggestion limiting our consumption of eggs must be considered arbitrary in the extreme. Eggs have been black listed because they contain cholesterol, but by what authority did those making such recommendations come to this conclusion? Were comparative studies conducted to assess the relative serum cholesterol levels over time in control groups eating no eggs, or eating just one egg, or two eggs, or ten eggs per week? Or, are these authorities self-ordained prophets who instinctively know a maximum of two or three eggs per week is the magic number? The answer to this question was made clear at a 1972 sitting of the United States National Commission on Egg Nutrition. Blandon Smith, the Chairman of the Commission, asked the Medical Director of the American Heart Foundation, Dr Campbell Moses, to cite the Foundation's scientific basis for recommending the consumption of eggs be limited to three each week. Doctor Moses replied that the Foundation's recommendation was based entirely on clinical opinion. At a subsequent sitting Dr Moses offered to stop mentioning eggs if the Commission would agree not to oppose the Heart Foundation's recommendation to limit cholesterol intake to 300 mg per day (United States Senate Select Committee on Foodstuffs, *Eggs and the AHA,* 10 September 1973). It is apparent that the American Heart Foundation's recommendation to limit cholesterol to a daily intake of 300 mg was also based on clinical opinion.

It is not uncommon to find nutritional recommendations in support of discarding the yolk of the egg in favour of the white, but this may create its own problem. The white of an egg contains avidin, a substance linked to skin eczema and body paralysis. But, the yolk of the egg contains a substance called biotin, the biological counterpart of avidin. When consumed together, the avidin in the white, and the biotin in the yolk, bind one to the other and become neutralised or conjugated. There is no evidence to suggest how many egg whites a person would have to consume to initiate the onset of eczema or body paralysis, but it does stress the need for maintaining a natural balance in our diets and in our lives.

In a time of diminishing protein resources, the egg offers us a nutritionally balanced, easily digested, readily obtainable, prepacked and stable food source which under refrigeration will stay fresh for weeks. You can fry it, scramble it, boil it, poach it and use it in a vast array of dishes from custard tarts to quiche, and still preserve its nutritional value.

For those concerned with the future of the environment, chicken sheds could easily be designed to harness the methane gas from their faecal droppings and convert it into useable energy. Methane gas produced daily by cattle and chickens is posing considerable threat to the ozone layer of this planet, but essential protein food in the form of chickens and eggs could be mass produced in an environmentally friendly manner. This cost effective and relatively limitless nutritional resource may justifiably occupy a position of greater importance in the diets of future generations.

Eggs are nature's little vitamin pills, chock-full of body building protein and goodness. Unfounded conjecture aside, there is not one scrap of scientific evidence to suggest the eating of eggs is anything less than good for you. You may eat as many eggs as you want provided you do not exceed your optimum daily allowance of protein as suggested by the *Slim Forever* program.

grains, breakfast cereals and bread

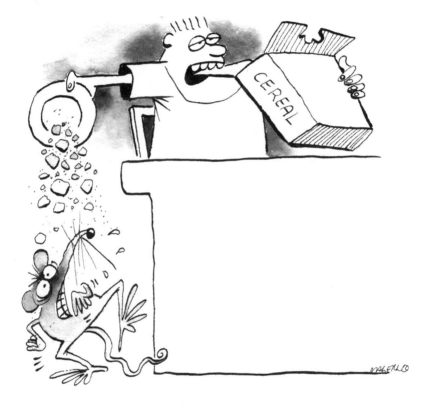

Grains

Breakfast cereals

Give us our daily bread

How important is fibre in the diet?

GRAINS

The humble grains have emerged from dietary obscurity to a position of domination. Grains did not become part of the human diet until our forebears made the transition from hunting to cultivating the soil. Our collective experience over the years has enabled us to grow grains commercially using hybrid strains to ensure higher yield. We now have the ability to grow grains in greater abundance than a world population of almost six billion people can consume.

Unlike highly perishable fruit, vegetable and meat products, grains are extremely stable and can be readily stored without refrigeration for indefinite periods. Grains are cost effective to produce and to transport and would make a wonderful food source, if only they were good for us.

Typically, a grain seed has a soft starchy centre called the endosperm which is covered by a thin layer of protective cellulose. Being starch, the centre of the grain is extremely low in nutrients but high in natural sugar — 50% to 80% in most cases. The outer cellulose covering and the reproductive germ of the grain contain most of the nutrients, but cellulose is indigestible to humans. Cellulose is the part of the grain we refer to as bulk or roughage which we are encouraged to eat to avoid constipation.

When grains are harvested they are nutritionally intact and contain some vitamins, minerals and incomplete protein, but the grain seldom goes directly from the field to the table. Most grains are stored before they are processed or sold and, as vitamins and minerals are relatively unstable, the nutrients in the grain readily break down. By the time most grains enter the processing stage much of their natural nutrients have been lost.

A large proportion of the grains we consume is in the form of flour, with a lesser portion going into the production of breakfast cereals.

How nutritious are grains?

Most of the nutrient content of any grain is in the outer cellulose casing and in the germ. Herbivores have the ability to digest cellulose and extract the vitamins, minerals and protein it contains, but not so humans. As cellulose is humanly indigestible, we absorb the abundance of sugar contained in the starch and pass most of the nutrients off in the faeces. The process of extracting and evaluating the nutritional content of grains in the laboratory is quite different to the process of human digestion.

The distribution of nutrients in grains becomes evident when rice is converted. Polished rice devoid of its cellulose outer layer is pure starch with no nutritional value. But, by parboiling the rice before it is polished some of the nutrients are driven out of the cellulose layer and into the starchy centre. This is a practice widely used in India where rice accounts for a large portion of the carbohydrate consumed in the daily diet.

Gluten intolerance from eating wheat, rye, oats and barley raises concern. Some individuals apparently lack the digestive enzyme necessary to hydrolyse gluten which leads to the onset of a condition known as non-tropical sprue or celiac disease. The gluten becomes toxic and attacks the lining of the intestine causing diarrhoea, weight loss, malaise and weakness. Anaemia, fluid retention and a tendency to intestinal bleeding may also occur. The secondary effects of gluten intolerance are impaired absorption of all nutrients, but especially fat, some protein, glucose, vitamins and calcium. Although many people are affected to a lesser degree and exhibit only mild symptoms usually not associated with gluten intolerance, estimates as to the incidence of this condition range as high as six out of every ten people.

BREAKFAST CEREALS

In the United States a Consumer Subcommittee of the Senate Committee on Commerce was convened in 1970 to inquire into the dry breakfast cereal industry. Robert B. Choate who was Chairman of the Council on Children in Washington D.C. appeared before that committee. He stated that of 60 commercial breakfast cereals tested for their protein, iron, calcium and vitamin content, 40 were rated as having no nutritional value. Choate also testified that laboratory tests involving rats fed a diet of ground up cereal boxes mixed with milk, sugar and raisins were healthier than rats fed on the cereals some of the boxes contained.

The dietary fibre revolution put gold in the hills for the breakfast cereal manufacturers who currently spend millions of dollars annually advertising their products. It obviously pays to advertise because most people now believe the eating of breakfast cereals is both nutritious and slimming.

The history of porridge and gruel dates back hundreds of years. Made from boiled grain, these inexpensive cereal dishes were a staple in prison diets and to the poor. However, the birth of the dry breakfast cereal industry as we know it did not occur until the 19th century. John Harvey Kellogg, a moralistic proponent of food reform, believed protein stimulated the sex drive which in turn lead to physical dissipation and exhaustion. Considering sexual activity to be an undesirable trait, he set about developing a carbohydrate breakfast cereal to replace the traditional breakfast of bacon and eggs. As protein is the only nutrient used in the generation of spermatozoa in the male and the formation of ova in the female, he may well have achieved his purpose.

Breakfast cereals are made by rolling various grains into flakes, or crushing and reconstituting them into appealing shapes. In all cases the process involves heat, and as most breakfast cereals are toasted, the extra heat employed is nutritionally catastrophic. In addition to the destruction of the 20 vitamins and minerals found naturally in grains, Dr Robert S. Goodhart of the New York Academy of Medicine and Dr Maurice E. Shils of the Cornell University Medical College suggest that the toasting of cereal products also decreases the physiological value of any natural protein the grain may have contained.

Toasting also removes or reduces the water content of the grain. Dehydration causes the remaining ingredients to become more concentrated, including the starch or sugar content of the grain. For example, fresh corn on the cob has a sugar content of 23% by weight, but cornflakes have a sugar content of 85%. Therefore, cornflakes are almost pure sugar. Now, add milk with a 5% sugar content, a spoon or two of cane sugar which is 100% pure sugar and you will have a breakfast of little more than sugar. If corn is your fancy you would do well to boil corn on the cob and add a little butter and sea salt. It will be better for you.

Children are targeted by cereal manufacturers who invade prime media viewing time with cartoons and advertisements urging children to request the purchase of their products. Children fare worse than adults when it comes to breakfast cereals with such sugar-added products as Froot Loops, Frosties and Coco Pops. Australian children are regularly confronted with a television commercial depicting a jovial tiger who tells them Frosties 'are greaaaaat mate', not withstanding that tigers are carnivores.

Choate's evidence to the Senate Subcommittee regarding the targeting of children by breakfast cereal manufacturers was damning.

He stated:

> *I believe our children are deliberately being sold the sponsor's*
> *less nutritious products over television. I believe our children are*
> *being programmed to demand sugar and sweetness in every food.*
> *I believe our children are being countereducated away from*
> *nutrition knowledge.*

Sugar is addictive, therefore the inducing of children to eat high sugar content breakfast cereals will ensure the ongoing purchase of those products.

GIVE US OUR DAILY BREAD

Bread has been referred to as the staff of life, but that was before the advent of modern production techniques. In the early days of milling, flour was produced by crushing the whole grain between stone rollers. The stone rollers were usually driven by wind, water or oxen power and moved slowly without generating heat. Vitamins and minerals are easily destroyed by heat, but the cold crushing techniques of times past guaranteed most of the nutrients, including the germ, were retained.

Not so today. Flour is milled by discarding the germ and the cellulose outer layer and crushing the grain between high speed steel rollers. Unlike the course ground whole grain flour produced by stone grinding, the flour we eat today is an extremely fine white powder. This the miller achieves by subjecting the grain to multiple crushing in a series of machines each with progressively finer roller settings. The heat generated by the steel rollers is capable of destroying any vitamins and minerals normally found in the grain, producing a finished product of lifeless off-white starch.

There are approximately 60 approved chemicals used in the making of flour and bread. Although no single manufacturer uses all 60 additives, eight or more are common place. For example, fresh flour is less than snow white and has a strong odour. To overcome these marketing deterrents the flour is gassed in special ovens using chlorine dioxide. The chlorine not only bleaches and matures the flour, it forms compounds such as dichlorostearic acid which remain in the flour. Chlorine dioxide destroys vitamin E, and reacts with certain proteins to form methionine sulfoxide which is known to cause central nervous system damage in humans. If chlorine dioxide is not used, bleaches such as benzoyl peroxide and nitrogen peroxide may be added together with maturing agents such as potassium bromate, potassium iodate and azocarbonamide.

Bread made from fresh stone ground flour is heavy and prone to drying and crumbling, a characteristic not desirable in today's commercially produced bread. Bakers are able to keep their product moist by adding polyoxyethlene monostearate which has the property of absorbing and retaining water. Water retention in the flour causes the bread to stand up and remain soft, but this chemical also causes cancer in laboratory rats. Ethoxylated mono- and diglycerides are also added to produce the desirable quality of softness in bread.

Fermentation is an important part of bread making. The addition of yeast causes the starch cells to rupture and the dough to rise, but the process of natural fermentation is too slow for commercial bakers. A fermentation accelerator is added in the form of ammonium chloride, a chemical compound also used in the manufacture of antifreeze for cars, and washing powder.

The more air holes there are in a loaf of bread the less flour it contains, and this is an important point in baking economics. A process developed in England and used widely throughout the industrialised world successfully combines the fermentation and aeration processes. This is achieved by adding 75 parts per million of potassium bromate and potassium iodate and mechanically whipping the dough. The dough becomes aerated and the fermentation time is reduced from between four and seven hours to just two minutes. Potassium bromate is a substance commonly found in home permanent hair wave products. Potassium iodate is known to cause gastrointestinal distress and the destruction of red blood cells when administered to test animals.

Milled white flour stripped of its natural inhibitors is extremely vulnerable to mould infestation. This is overcome by adding propionic acid, the anti-fungal ingredient in athletes foot powder.

Do you prefer wholemeal bread? Wholemeal bread is made from white flour to which is added chemically treated wheat germ. Doris Grant, author of *Your Daily Food,* suggests the addition of chemically treated wheat germ makes the finished product twice as harmful as bread made from white flour alone.

'Enriched', 'hi-fibre' and 'fibre-added' are terms appearing on many bread wrappers, but what do they mean? During the course of manufacture the bread we buy is denuded of all 20 natural vitamins and minerals and what little protein the grain originally contained. Bakers add an average of just three or four synthetic vitamins and minerals and claim their product to be enriched. In the absence of the other 16 or 17 nutrients destroyed in the milling process, the term 'degraded' may be more appropriate.

'Hi-fibre' and 'fibre-added' suggest the bread you are buying will assist in keeping you regular. There is no fibre in starch, so the bakers add non-digestible vegetable fibre or synthetic methyl cellulose to replace the fibre contained in the discarded cellulose shell.

HOW IMPORTANT IS FIBRE IN THE DIET?

Dietary fibre assists in the digestion and absorption process of the food we eat, but our need for fibre has been grossly overstated. Fibre is vegetable matter consisting of indigestible polysaccharides, cellulose and gums which are also found in fruit, vegetables and in the outer casing of grains.

Fibre acts by mixing with, and adding bulk to the food bolus as it moves through the intestine. The contents of the intestine are moved forward by peristalsis, an action initiated by the rhythmic contractions of tiny muscles in the wall of the intestine. The stimulation of peristalsis is to some degree initiated by the degrading action of bacteria on digestible carbohydrate. But, as cellulose is indigestible it does not promote bacterial action and may actually contribute to constipation, not prevent it. Doctor James M. Orten of Wayne State University School of Medicine and Doctor Otto W. Neuhaus of the University of South Dakota School of Medicine state that while food must contain fibre, an abundance of fibre tends to produce constipation.

The peristaltic action also churns the food bolus over and over in an effort to bring the nutrients in contact with the absorptive surface of the intestine. If the food bolus is too sloppy, the contents cannot be successfully churned and the food will quickly pass through the body. A food bolus which is too dry, or food containing too much fibre, will also resist the churning action of peristalsis, and again nutrient absorption will be impaired.

The consumption of the cellulose covering of grains causes yet another problem. During the mastication process our teeth fracture the cellulose outer covering on the grain before it is swallowed. Grain cellulose is constructed of millions of tiny, but very hard, closed cells which make it relatively impervious to water. As cellulose cannot absorb water it passes through the intestine as it was swallowed, but the sharp edges left from chewing act as tiny razors on the villi of the intestine. This position is supported by Dr Orten and Dr Neuhaus who suggest an overabundance of fibre can lead to irritation of the intestinal mucosa. A standard procedure in treating peptic ulcers is the removal of fibre from the diet, further evidence as to the ability of some fibre to irritate the sensitive lining of the intestinal tract.

The water-resistant quality of cellulose is the reason why whole grains have to be pre-softened with chemicals before they can be included in the bread baking process.

How much fibre should I eat?

The need for fibre in a balanced diet, although absolutely essential, is relatively low. However, diets high in processed flour products lack the natural bulk found in fruit and vegetables. If you take a slice of white bread and soak it in a saucer of water it will quickly turn to slime, and this is exactly what it does in your intestine. Diets high in processed carbohydrates, such as bread, cake, cookies and buns, require additional fibre from other carbohydrate foods, all of which contain natural or added sugar. The consumption of concentrated dietary fibre in drink and food-added forms is testimony in support of our poor eating habits.

If you are seeking a healthier and more regular life pattern you would do well to concentrate on reducing your sugar and starch intake by limiting the quantity of processed grain products you consume. Processed cereal grains, white flour and products made from white flour have little to offer of nutritional value and are a poor choice of dietary fibre. Vegetables of the green and yellow varieties are relatively high in vitamins and minerals and contain soft indigestible polysaccharides and cellulose ideally suited to aiding human digestion.

Once your system responds to a balance of foods as outlined in your *Slim Forever* program, a diet of protein with a salad, or two or three vegetables each day will produce a food bolus of exactly the correct consistency. Your intestine will not be filled with excessive amounts of indigestible fibre, and the absorption rate of nutrients contained in the food will be enhanced.

sugar 'n' spice and everything ...?

16

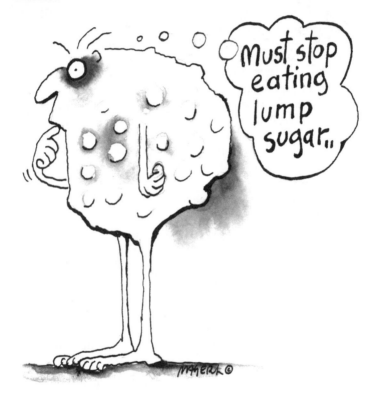

Where does all the sugar go?

Why do we eat so much sugar?

Why is sugar so harmful?

How much sugar is too much?

Sugar was introduced to the industrialised world in the late eighteenth century by traders plying the West Indies. Considered a spice, sugar was expensive and only the rich were able to afford a light sprinkle on their fruit pies. Not so today. Our daily consumption of sugar is 25 times greater than it was 200 years ago. Now, every man, woman and child in the industrialised world is consuming in the vicinity of 120 lb/55 kg of refined sugar each year. This frightening statistic means many individuals are consuming the equivalent of their own body weight in refined sugar every 12 months.

We are at risk of sugar dominating our diets, but our addiction to sugar goes way beyond eating it. Sugar has even impacted our vocabulary. We use the implication of sweetness as being good and to describe all things beautiful. We commonly use such phrases as 'hi sugar', 'sweet dreams', 'isn't she sweet', 'my sweetheart', 'sweeten the deal', 'home sweet home', and 'don't sugar coat it, give it to me straight'. Even the great one, Jackie Gleason, made famous his signature line 'how sweet it is'.

We tend to think of the sugar we consume as the granulated white crystals we sprinkle on our breakfast cereal and add to our tea or coffee. If that was all we ate there would be little problem, but like hidden fats in manufactured food, it is the sugar we cannot see that does the damage. Sugar is added in incredible quantities to almost every processed food we consume, but let us not just blame the food manufacturers. Manufactured food is becoming increasingly sweeter because we the consumers demand it be sweeter. Like any addiction our craving for sugar has become self-perpetuating. The more we eat, the more we want.

WHERE DOES ALL THE SUGAR GO?

Sugar is used extensively in the manufacture of soft drinks, chocolate, candy, cakes, cookies and ice-cream. But, it is also added to such items as manufactured meat products, yoghurt, peanut butter, jams, jellies, bread, sauces, ketchup and gravy mixes. Some naturally high sugar content fruit varieties such as peaches, apricots and pineapple often have sugar added during the preserving process. Even canned and frozen vegetables such as peas, carrots and beans can be the targets of refined sugar during packaging. Yoghurt, a biologically active food of relatively low sugar content in its natural state, is almost unrecognisable in its marketed sugar and flavour-added form. Yet, sweetened yoghurt is consumed daily by millions of people in the misguided belief that it is good for them, and will help them lose unwanted body fat.

The soft drink industry is the largest user of sugar in the world. The average can of soft drink contains 8 teaspoons of sugar with some drinks as high as 17 teaspoons of sugar. A can of regular Coca-Cola contains 1.4 oz /39.75 g of added sugar which is enough to supply a person of 145 lb/65 kg lean body weight with sufficient carbohydrate to last 18 hours. People with an addiction to Coca-Cola may drink as many as one or two dozen cans each day, consuming enough carbohydrate to last a person of average build from nine to 18 days.

The chocolate, candy and ice-cream industries are next on the list of major sugar users. The Swiss and the British are the world champion chocolate eaters, with every man, woman and child consuming an average of 28 lb/12.5 kg of chocolate each year. The United States outshines the world when it comes to eating ice-cream with an average annual per capita consumption of $5\frac{1}{2}$ gal/25 L. But, the Swiss and the British eat almost as much ice-cream as the North Americans who in turn eat almost as much chocolate as their European counterparts.

The major component in most chocolate and candy is refined cane or beet sugar. A 2 oz/60 g Mars bar, which we are told will fill the gap before dinner, has a total sugar content of 1.45 oz/41 g. More than filling the gap, a Mars a day will supply enough sugar to keep the average sized person in carbohydrate for at least 19 hours.

Maryon Stewart in her book *Beat Sugar Craving* offers some very interesting statistics regarding the consumption of confectionery. Women buy 65% of all candy and chocolate, while men buy 27%, and children under the age of 14 years buy 8%. Of all confectionery manufactured women consume 39%, children under 14 years consume 35%, while men consume

26%. Perhaps the most significant statistic relates to children under the age of 14 years who eat four times more confectionery than they buy, which means they get most of it from their mothers.

WHY DO WE EAT SO MUCH SUGAR?

We are trained from infancy to eat sugar. Mothers buy manufactured prepared baby food in the belief it is wholesome. In the 1980s a major baby food manufacturer in the United States was prosecuted for selling a product labelled fruit juice which proved to be sugar and water with synthetic flavour, but no fruit juice. Even unlikely manufactured infant meals such as strained meat and vegetables sometimes contain added sugar. Manufactured baby food may also contain approved preservatives from the nitrate group, and sodium carboxymethyl cellulose.

Babies are often given bread sticks to suck which are approximately 50% sugar in the form of starch. And, junior's dummy or pacifier is often dipped in something sweet as an inducement for the child to keep sucking instead of crying. *Lancet* (12 June 1969) published the results of a survey conducted at the Paediatric Unit of St Mary's Hospital in London. Two out of every three mothers surveyed admitted adding sweeteners to their baby's bottle.

When baby is able to consume solid food many parents delight in giving them treats such as toast with jam or jelly, sugar-added drinks, cake, cookies, candy, chocolate and ice-cream. Many children start their day by eating a naturally high sugar content breakfast cereal to which they add yet more refined sugar. Or, perhaps they choose a highly sugar-added breakfast cereal such as Coco Pops, Froot Loops or Frosties. Add to this white bread for toast and sandwiches, flavoured milk, a soft drink, a candy bar, an ice-cream, a slice of cake and a handful of cookies, and their day is complete. It is little wonder people reach adulthood with programmed insatiable appetites for sugar, a substance perhaps no less addictive to some than alcohol, nicotine and certain drugs.

WHY IS SUGAR SO HARMFUL?

Sugar is not harmful if we consume it in limited quantities as it occurs naturally in our diet. But, highly concentrated sugar extracted from cane and beet is quite a different story. Cane and beet sugars consumed to excess have the ability to:

- depress the burning of body fat for energy;

- cause the conditions of being overweight and obesity;

- cause dental decay;

- initiate the onset of diabetes mellitus;

- depress the production of white blood cells and the effectiveness of the auto-immune system;

- precipitate headaches; and

- lower the body's pain threshold.

Sucrose does occur naturally in our food chain but it took human ingenuity to extract and crystallise a juice so potent it can adversely affect and even shorten our lives. John Yudkin, Emeritus Professor of Nutrition at Queen Elizabeth College, London University, and the author of a book on sugar entitled, *Pure White and Deadly,* advocates a total government ban on the sale of refined sugar.

Advanced agricultural methods have also contributed to our addiction to sugar. Coupled with our ability to graft and create new and sweeter varieties of fruit is our increasing tendency to choose fruit according to its sugar content. The sweeter the fruit, the better we like it. Modern refrigeration, improved transportation and artificial ripening techniques have also contributed to our addiction to sugar. Unseasonal fruit such as tropical bananas and papaya can now be enjoyed by the people of Iceland in the middle of winter. And, cold weather fruit such as apples are available in the Pacific islands in the middle of summer. Perhaps a lack of variety and a level of boredom born of more of the same in times past may have been more a health benefit than an inconvenience.

HOW MUCH SUGAR IS TOO MUCH?

Although small quantities of carbohydrate qualify as an essential ingredient in our daily diet, we did not develop as predominantly sugar eaters. Our metabolic systems are simply not capable of handling the large quantities of refined sugar we are currently consuming, and we are paying the price with our health and our lives. Even a lean person of very large stature has an optimum daily carbohydrate requirement of only 3 oz/90 g, a quantity too many people consume at breakfast. As our bodies do not differentiate between sources of carbohydrate, the sugar from a piece of chocolate will behave exactly the same as sugar from fruit and vegetables. But, as chocolate, candy, soft drinks and ice-cream are non-foods largely devoid of vitamins and minerals, a person deriving his or her carbohydrate needs from such sources may be nutritionally deficient. Many obese people suffer malnutrition because they eat enormous quantities of lifeless, fattening food. For example, one can of Coca-Cola and one Mars bar have a combined sugar content of 2.85 oz/81 g. This is the sugar equivalent of up to 17 lb/8 kg of artichokes, asparagus, aubergine (egg plant), avocado, broccoli, brussels sprouts, cabbage, capsicum (bell peppers), carrots, cauliflower, celery, french beans, lettuce, marrow, pumpkin, rhubarb, spinach and tomatoes.

Fortunately, our bodies allow us leeway to realise some of our food fantasies without gaining unwanted body fat. Using the above examples, 2.85 oz/81 g of sugar contained in one can of Coca-Cola and a Mars bar is the *Slim Forever* weight maintenance allowance for a person with a lean body weight of 210 lb/96 kg. Although large of stature, a person of this size is unlikely to consume 17 lb/8 kg of vegetables in a day. Nor does he or she need to. A moderate serve of just three vegetables, or a fresh garden salad made from a variety of vegetables will supply any person with all the vitamins, minerals and fibre necessary for good health. The balance of the carbohydrate allowance can be used to consume any other food that may tickle one's fancy, provided the sum of the carbohydrates does not exceed 80 g.

Why do we become addicted to sugar?

Once sugar enters the human digestive system it has but one path to follow. The fate of all sugar is the synthesis of glucose, and the sole purpose of glucose is the production of energy. The blood in our system passes through the pancreas where the sugar it contains signals the need for the production of the hormone insulin. Insulin is produced by the beta cells of the pancreas and released into the blood where it attaches itself to the glucose. Glucose can only produce energy if it is inside a tissue cell, but its size precludes entry into the cell without the assistance of insulin. Glucose which is surplus to the immediate requirements of the cells remains in the bloodstream, and under the influence of insulin it is later absorbed by the liver and fat cells and converted into body fat.

The player to watch here is not glucose, but insulin. Peculiar to most body functions is a slight lag in time between generating the signal, and the commencement of the desired function. In the case of glucose, the sugar must be in the blood before a response for the production of insulin can be initiated. A person eating food with a high sugar content creates a rush of glucose in the blood and becomes temporarily hyperglycaemic. High blood sugar signals the need for high insulin production and the pancreas is forced into action to the limit of its manufacturing capabilities. However, there is also a lag in time between the pancreas sensing a drop in serum glucose levels and a corresponding reduction in the volume of insulin being produced. Under balanced dietary conditions we maintain a level of glucose in the blood, free of the effects of insulin, to be used for the production of energy in an emergency. But, the time lag between the pancreas sensing a drop in the presence of glucose and ceasing insulin production results in overproduction. The additional insulin produced has no option other than to seek out the emergency supplies of serum glucose and drag it off into the cells. This in turn causes an abnormal drop in serum glucose levels and the onset of a condition known as hypoglycaemia. Low blood sugar signals the hunger response, but extreme low blood sugar associated with hypoglycaemia causes a person to feel light-headed and faint, with a craving for something sweet to eat.

Known as the hyper-hypoglycaemic swing this seesawing effect between excessively high and excessively low blood sugar keeps the tissue cells filled to capacity with glucose. Instead of drawing upon fat reserves for the production of the major portion of energy, the body develops a preference for low-energy sugar. This results in energy being produced almost entirely from glucose to the exclusion of fat. Existing body fat is retained while additional fat is constantly being formed from the excess of serum glucose.

Under balanced dietary conditions the rise and fall in blood sugar is so mild the effects of the two extremes are not consciously felt. When normal levels of blood sugar are maintained the tissue cells are free to draw on energy-ready triglycerides from the fat storage cells, and the overall level of body fat will decrease. Once a desired level of fat loss is achieved, a balanced diet will create a state of equilibrium between the formation and degradation of body fat. As the amount of fat formation will now equal the amount of fat used for the production of energy, the formation of unwanted body fat will never again be an issue.

Sugar and diabetes mellitus

Yet another problem arises from the over-consumption of sugar. Unable to sustain high volume insulin production, and under constant pressure from incoming sugar, the beta cells of the pancreas will in time simply wear out. With little or no insulin produced internally, the body suffers uncontrolled hyperglycaemia and the onset of diabetes mellitus.

One Australian in every 25 suffers from diagnosed diabetes mellitus. Perhaps even more frightening are the estimates suggesting one person in every two is a borderline diabetic, a damning legacy of excessive sugar consumption. Doctor John Carter, President of the Australian Diabetes Society, stated that four Australians an hour develop diabetes in a country with a population of less than 17 million. According to Dr Carter diabetes is one of the single largest causes of death in Australia. It predisposes heart attacks, strokes and kidney failure, and is the most common cause of blindness in adults over 65 years of age (*Sunday Telegraph,* 30 May 1993).

However, a number of borderline and insulin-dependent diabetics have, without exception, responded positively to the *Slim Forever* program. Insulin-dependent diabetics, under the supervision of the author, have been able to totally cease the taking of all medication and have displayed normal serum glucose levels within one or two days of commencing this program.

WARNING

If you are an insulin dependent diabetic, consult with your physician before undertaking any dietary change, including changes outlined in this text. Alterations in diet, or in the dosage of insulin without prior medical advice, could result in the onset of either insulin shock or diabetic coma.

Sugar and heart disease

Diabetes mellitus and heart disease were not considered major killers 100 years ago when sugar was consumed in much smaller quantities. Although medical science claims mastery over many diseases, the average life span over the past 75 years has only risen from 70 to 72 years. This suggests that while lives are being saved with advances in science in many areas, a negative and deadly force is opposing increases in overall longevity. This deadly force may well be sugar.

Professor Yudkin reports an increase in the number of people diagnosed as suffering from heart disease among European communities consuming higher than average quantities of refined sugar.

Diabetes and heart disease are unknown to the members of the Masai nation in Africa. But, when removed from their natural habitat these people suffer diabetes and heart disease equally with their industrialised neighbours. The traditional Masai diet consists of milk and animal blood, contrasting significantly with their adopted urban diets which contain large quantities of processed and highly refined carbohydrates.

The evidence is clear, refined sugar has no place in our diets. If you are concerned about your weight and your health, avoid refined sugar and all foods which contain refined sugar. You will be amazed how good you will feel without it.

what have they done to our food?

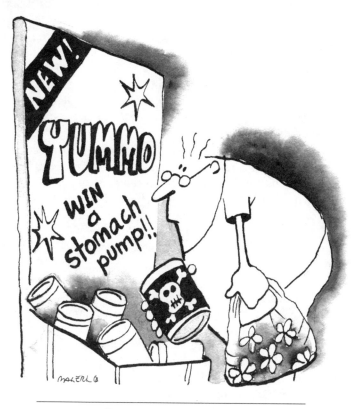

Nature provided us with 103 elementary chemicals. Modern science has managed to produce greater than 60,000 chemical concoctions, approximately 6,000 of which are used directly in growing and processing the food we eat.

There can be little doubt as to the deleterious impact these hybrid chemical compounds are having on our fragile environment. Over the past 50 years we have succeeded in poisoning our land, our rivers and our oceans. We have polluted the air we breathe, and we have played a major role in bringing about the extinction of many life forms native to this planet. We bear witness to an increase in the incidence of diagnosed cancer and other chemically induced diseases in plants, animals and humans. Yet, we persist with our roller-coaster ride of chemical self-destruction.

High profile groups demonstrably oppose the destruction we are wreaking upon our environment, but we are doing little to oppose the addition of chemicals to the food we eat. Acting in their own self-interest, many food manufacturers have seized upon our excusable ignorance of scientific fact. Contemptibly, they contrive to conceal or down play the harmful effects chemical food additives are having on our health and well-being.

Governments have sold out by permitting the adoption of a numerical coding system to replace the specific names of chemicals listed on food labels. The human brain has the capacity to commit to memory the individual names and related functions of these various chemicals. But, the committing to memory of thousands of multi-digit numbers together with the name and function of the chemical each number represents is almost impossible. The official reasons given for the adoption of the numerical chemical system are:

- international standardisation; and

- the saving of space on food wrappers.

Given that most governments require imported food to be labelled in the language of the importing country, the use of numbers in place of names cannot be justified. And, as small quantities of food are often packaged in large containers to gain greater shelf advertising space, the assertion of being space saving fails the credibility test. Some local health authorities offer a free pamphlet listing a number of the most common food additives by both name and number, but the list is typically far from complete. These pamphlets are but a token gesture of governmental concern, as the probability of shoppers screening supermarket shelves with booklet in hand is remote.

The list of approved food additives is frightening. Boasting over 2,000 the list includes substances such as:

■ carbon and iron oxide blacks;

■ hydrochloric and phosphoric acids;

■ potassium ferrocyanide;

■ aluminium silicates and phosphates;

■ benzoyl peroxide; and

■ ethyl alcohol.

It also includes non-foods such as bees wax, and a chalky substance known as kaolin which is used to make talcum powder. In a touch of irony the additive gelatine which is made from natural protein and appears as number 441 is being removed from the list. Any processed food using this natural substance is now required to state the name 'gelatine' in full on the label. The legislated disclosure of the full names of natural additives while toxic substances hide behind an innocuous numbering system is nothing short of pandering.

Bugs in agriculture

Agricultural science continues to develop new and stronger chemicals for use in the production of food. Overplanting leaches the soil of its nutrients, demanding replacement by the application of fertilisers in ever increasing amounts. The widespread use of pesticides has resulted in the selective breeding of more resilient bugs by killing the weak and leaving only the strong to multiply. More potent chemical pesticides are constantly being developed in an effort to stop these superbugs from eating our food before we do. All good news for the grower but bad news for the consumer. Or is it?

The abuse of chemical additives in agriculture is starting to take a toll on productivity. There is growing evidence of a trend towards lower agricultural yield, diminished product size and shorter shelf life of perishable produce. The process has come full circle, but, there is some good news. Some farmers in Europe and Great Britain have adopted a no chemical approach to growing produce. Almost immediate increases in yield with better product size and longer shelf life have been reported. In the absence of agricultural chemicals there has been a welcomed return of bugs which do not eat the product but eat the bugs that do. Mother Nature in her infinite wisdom created balance and harmony among all things. It has taken us less than 50 years to significantly upset that delicate balance, a balance which has been billions of years in the making.

CHEMICALS IN OUR FOOD

The rapid spoilage rate of food, especially food of animal origin, spurred the development of yet another range of chemicals in the form of preservatives. Food spoilage occurs when perishable food is exposed to the air, and the bacteria it contains. Bacteria invade the defenceless food and quickly multiply, causing the food to putrefy. By creating an environment which is poisonous to the invading bacteria, putrefaction can be controlled. But, at what cost?

Bacteria fall into two distinct categories of being either humanly friendly, or unmistakably unfriendly. Approximately 85% of all species of bacteria are humanly friendly, with many living permanently in our intestines as flora. These friendly little critters undertake the very important task of converting any residual post-digestive food bolus into faecal material prior to defecation. The remaining 15% of bacteria are the bad guys. These unfriendly bacteria are capable of making us ill and in some cases of even causing death. However, killing them with chemical food additives is definitely not the answer. Chemicals such as sodium nitrate, sodium nitrite, sodium erythorbate, butylated-hydroxyanisole (BHA) and butylated-hydroxytoluene

(BHT) will kill most bacteria on contact. But, these chemicals are absorbed full strength into our digestive tracts where they set about killing our friendly and essential bacteria as well. Losing flora in the intestine would be enough by itself, but these chemicals also find their way into the bloodstream. And that is where the real damage is done.

Our bodies have no natural defence against these man-made chemicals. As they did not form part of our developmental environment, our systems were not required to develop a barrier against their absorption. Nor was it required to develop an effective method of neutralising these chemicals once they are inside the body. Chemicals in the bloodstream either find their way into the living tissue cells, or into the fat storage cells where they may lay dormant for years.

TOXIC CHEMICALS VERSUS LIVING TISSUE

Each living cell contains an operating code in the form of a strand of interlocking commands known as deoxyribonucleic acid (DNA). The detail on the DNA strand gives each cell its individuality, but the sequence of coding can be changed. For example, if the DNA strand of a liver cell was totally replaced with a DNA strand from a kidney cell, the liver cell would function as a kidney cell. However, total transplants do not occur in nature, but partial alterations to the individual commands on the strands do. If a coding system is altered in any way, the host cell will change function accordingly. But, more importantly, it will pass the altered code sequence on to its progeny. Alterations usually occur when a foreign substance such as radiation, infection or a toxic chemical displaces part of the code. In cases of chemical toxicity the chemical itself may attach itself to the vacant site on the strand.

Every cell has a predetermined life span of between a few hours and four months. Some cells in the eye have a life span of only two or three hours, but the great survivor is the red blood cell with a life span of 120 days. When a cell reaches the end of its programmed life it builds a replacement cell by constructing a sequel to its DNA strand. The strands separate and the sequel DNA creates a new cell in the exact likeness of the old cell. The expired cell disintegrates and the debris is carried away by the bloodstream. Known as mitosis, this innate ability of cells to replicate is the source of life, but it is also the reason we age. Damage to a cell's DNA strand does not heal and the imprint of that damage is passed on to all future generations of cells. The accumulative effect of these minute alterations takes its toll and in time the body will begin to show signs of ageing. However, we can do something positive about the ageing process by avoiding all, or any of the cell damaging elements.

Enter the toxic chemicals

Once a cell absorbs a toxic chemical it renders its DNA strand vulnerable to attack. If the chemical manages to implant itself on the strand, the DNA code will be altered and the function of the cell will change accordingly. But, as the change does not usually conform with any other biological coding in the body, the cell becomes a mutant or cancer cell. Mutant cells lose the discipline of healthy cells. The ability to replicate is retained by the mutant cell, however, the obligatory life span is no longer imposed. In consequence the mutant cell and its progeny continue to propagate but refuse to die.

Each organ in the body has the ability to control both its size and shape by regulating the number of cells it contains. Known as touch inhibition, this mechanism enables the organ to produce no more or less cells than are required, and to maintain the cells in an orderly pattern. Mutant cells do not possess the touch inhibition factor and will continue to multiply unchecked. Now, as healthy cells are unable to differentiate between functional and mutant cells, they register the presence of mutant cells as if they were functional cells. If the correct number of cells are perceived to be present a healthy cell will disintegrate without initiating the replication process. This results in the uncontrolled multiplication of mutant cells and the diminished presence of functional cells.

The relative uniformity of size of each healthy cell is another factor not shared by mutant cells. With no specific function to perform, the mutants engorge nutrients and grow to enormous sizes. Ageless existence, size, and the absence of touch inhibition soon combine and the mutant cells eventually overtake the host organ.

Functional cells are very stable in their environment, unlike some mutant cells which may break away and travel in the bloodstream. Known as metastasis, this process allows a mutant cell to relocate to another part of the body, there to resume its insane multiplication and growth pattern.

Are food chemicals to blame?

When fed to rats, a number of food preservatives such as sodium nitrate and sodium nitrite are known to be cancer-forming. The manufacturing industry cries foul and argues that the concentrations of chemicals fed to the test animals were in amounts far exceeding the concentrations found in processed food. Their argument indeed appears to be valid. But, while the concentration of preservatives in a particular food may be relatively low, the accumulative effect over time must also be considered. The annual per capita consumption of chemicals contained in processed food in the industrialised world exceeds 3 lb/1.4 kg. How concentrated do these chemicals have to be?

With a total consumption of around 216 lb/98 kg, most people consume greater than their body weight of often toxic food additives during the course of their life. Another point apparently overlooked by the processed food industry is that it takes just one molecule of a toxic chemical to affect one cell and set the mutation process in motion. Even if the chances of this happening are millions to one, the odds are significantly reduced every time a gram of toxic chemical is ingested.

Medical science is striving to find a cure for cancer, but in this case an ounce of prevention may well be better than a pound of cure. Instead of spending huge sums of money on research, surely it makes more sense to remove as many known causes of this dreaded disease from our environment as is possible. The eradication of unnecessary chemical additives to our food would be a giant step in the right direction.

THE ART OF DECEPTION

Many of the chemicals used in the manufacture of food have been grouped under less offensive names in an obvious attempt to placate the buying public.

These groups include:

- *anti-caking agents* which are added to ensure products such as salt flow freely when poured;

- *bleaching agents* used to lighten the colour of food such as flour and cooking oils;

- *anti-oxidants* which prevent food containing fats and oils from becoming rancid;

- *emulsifiers* which are added to ensure oil and water mixtures do not separate, and to ensure moisture does not form fragments of ice in frozen food;

- *artificial colourings* added to heighten or restore natural colour lost during refinement and to ensure uniformity of colour;

- *flavour enhancers* to magnify the flavour of the food without imparting a flavour of their own;

- *mineral salts* added to enhance the texture of processed meats and to prevent the loss of fat and natural juices during cooking;

- *preservatives* designed to prolong the shelf life of food by retarding bacterial infestation;

- *humectants* added to prevent food from drying out; and

- *thickeners and vegetable gums* which ensure uniform consistency in the product.

If food in its natural state requires chemical additives to preserve it, make it pour more freely, bleach it, colour it, emulsify it, flavour it, moisturise and thicken it, all before we eat it, one can only wonder where nature went wrong.

You may be astonished to learn of the alternative uses of some of the additives found in our processed food. For example, the emulsifier diethyl glucol added to commercial ice-cream to prevent ice formation is anti-freeze, the very same chemical you put in the radiator of your car. To overcome the problem of raw potato chips and french fries going brown before cooking, the product is washed in a diluted solution of difluorodichloromethane. Also known as Freon 12, the refrigerant, difluorodichloromethane is a close relative of white spirit used in the dry cleaning of clothes and in the manufacture of paint stripper.

IS MEDICATION SAFE?

No treatise on chemicals in food would be complete without making reference to prescription and non-prescription medication. Like most industries, our health care industry is profit driven, and it profits the drug manufacturing companies to be able to offer a chemical cure for every known ailment. But, is the cost limited to the purchase price of the medication?

The giant strides claimed by medical science are being overshadowed by the emergence of new and more powerful diseases in almost plague proportions. The 1980s saw the emergence of the killer AIDS virus, and in 1992 a new, more deadly and drug resistant strain of tuberculosis appeared on the scene. In 1993 a new and more virulent strain of cholera was detected. Influenza is no longer a two day inconvenience. Each year the strains of influenza virus appear to be stronger than in previous years, and lives are being claimed. Like the super bugs in our fields which developed in response to more and stronger insecticides, the role of prescription drugs in the emergence of drug resistant strains of infection cannot be discounted.

The validity of multiple prescription drug taking must also be questioned. Few chemicals are stable in the presence of other chemicals and most will interact to produce a chemical compound quite different from the original compounds. Preliminary results from studies currently under way in the United States indicate a ratio as high as one in three aged persons may be dying prematurely from the toxic effects of multiple drug taking. This finding is corroborated by a recent Australian study which revealed that one in every three aged people were taking multiple prescription drugs. The coincidence cannot be ignored.

An excerpt from a paper issued in 1979 by the United States Department of Health, Education and Welfare entitled 'Healthy people: The Surgeon General's report on health promotion and disease prevention' stated: "You the individual can do more for your own health and well-being than any doctor, any hospital, any drug, any exotic medical advice." Good advice indeed. It may take a little more than an apple a day to keep the doctor away. But, in the face of more potent diseases and soaring health costs, a balanced diet free of toxic chemicals together with a daily regimen of moderate exercise makes very good sense.

IS THERE AN ALTERNATIVE?

Yes. For every chemical additive used in the manufacture and processing of food, a more natural and non-toxic alternative is available. Industry would have us believe the healthy alternatives are more expensive, and would add to the cost of the finished product. But, as with all manufacturing techniques, the more a process is used the cheaper it becomes. By alerting ourselves to the effects toxic chemicals have on our bodies, and by refusing to purchase chemically contaminated food, we can collectively pressure industry into changing its manufacturing agenda.

18

biorhythms
and
biological clocks

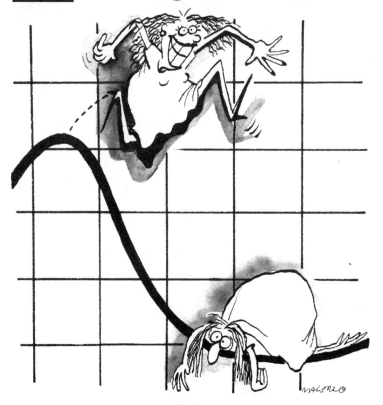

Biorhythms

The 24-hour biological clock

BIORHYTHMS

The universe contains millions of planets and stars which are made of gas and solid matter. The order of these astrological bodies is maintained by an immense energy source, and we as individuals are an extension of that source.

Energy does not travel in a straight line. Energy moves in a strict wave pattern, alternately rising above and dipping below a line of neutrality. Like the universal energy that influences us, our energy patterns also rise and fall in a rhythmic pattern of life. These patterns of energy are referred to as biorhythms.

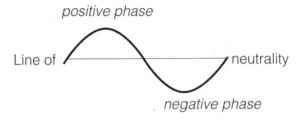

A Typical Wave Pattern
Figure 18.1

Biorhythmic energy

Our lives are governed by three energy sources, namely:

- the source of physical energy;

- the source of emotional energy; and

- the source of intellectual energy.

In the late nineteenth century Dr Hermann Swoboda who was Professor of Psychology at the University of Vienna, and a physician in Berlin named Dr William Fliess, were independently researching apparent changes in physical and emotional energy. They each discovered that individuals displayed alterations in energy levels according to a time scale, with corresponding periods of high and low energy. The time occupied by an increase in energy was precisely equal to the length of time occupied by a decrease in energy in all individuals. This led to the conclusion that our energy is governed by a wave pattern which rises and falls in a similar fashion to the universal energy which surrounds us.

At the turn of the century, an Austrian engineer and teacher named Dr Alfred Teltscher observed the ability of students to concentrate. He discovered the intellectual capacity of each student strengthened and weakened equally over a given period of time, and repeated itself in exactly the same time frame. From these three men came the birth of our understanding of human biorhythms.

When do our biorhythms start functioning?

Our physical, emotional and intellectual biorhythms commence functioning at precisely the moment we start life outside of the uterus. Once initiated, these biorhythms function within us for the remainder of our lives. It is interesting to note that from the moment of birth all three biorhythms rise and remain in the positive phase for approximately the first two weeks of life. This is also the most critical period of life when we strive to establish our existence independently of our mothers.

How do biorhythms differ?

Our physical, emotional and intellectual biorhythms differ in both wave length and effect. Our physical biorhythm spans a period of 23 days with 11½ days of high physical energy and 11½ days of low physical energy. Our emotional biorhythm has a span of 28 days with 14 days of high emotional energy and 14 days of low emotional energy. And, the intellectual biorhythm, which is the longest of the three, has a span of 33 days with 16½ days of high intellectual activity and 16½ days of low intellectual activity.

The physical biorhythm

When your physical biorhythm is in the positive phase you will experience a feeling of heightened physical well-being. Your

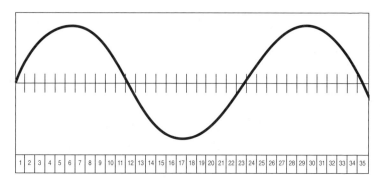

The physical biorhythm

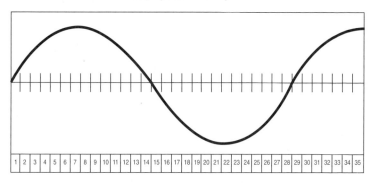

The emotional biorhythm

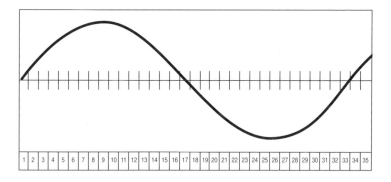

The intellectual biorhythm

The Wave Lengths of Biorhythms
Figure 18.2

days will be more energetic, your muscles will feel firmer, and you will be able to sustain longer and more intense periods of physical activity. Athletes typically perform better during the positive phase of their physical biorhythm, often recording their best efforts.

As your physical biorhythm dips into the negative phase your energy level will progressively fall until you reach the lowest point of the arc. You will perform below your peak physical ability, you will tire more quickly and you will require more sleep. Your muscles will lose a degree of tone and may ache slightly when subjected to heavy exercise. You can take advantage of your physical cycle by planning more intense physical activities to coincide with the positive phase of this biorhythm.

Although the negative phase of your physical biorhythm occupies $11\frac{1}{2}$ days of the total cycle, your period of poorest physical activity usually lasts only five days. This period commences two days before and extends three days after the moment when your physical biorhythm reaches its lowest ebb on the negative arc. Once your physical biorhythm enters the fourth day of its upward swing you will feel energy returning to your body. But, you will not experience a return to maximum energy until the biorhythm crosses the line of neutrality. In effect you will have approximately 12 days of high energy, six days of acceptable energy and five days of low energy. If you exercise regularly you should maximise your efforts during the positive and transition periods as these are your times of greatest potential improvement. For the five day period of poor physical ability you should rest, re-energise your body and undertake only light maintenance exercise. This is not a good time to climb a mountain or clean the garage. You will quickly fatigue.

The emotional biorhythm

For a period of 14 days out of every 28 you will be at your emotional and creative best. This is your period of greatest need for sharing and being in the company of others. It is a time when you will be most demonstrable with your affections and you will display your greatest emotional strength.

During the negative phase of this biorhythm you may display emotional indifference and feel slightly depressed. You will have greater need for demonstrated affection from others and you may seek overt confirmation of that affection. This is the period when you are given to asking, 'Do you still love me?'

To organise your life around the positive and negative phases of your emotional biorhythm would be an impossible task. You do not choose to fall in love according to a time schedule, nor can you organise your moments of excitement or despair to coincide with the positive phase of your emotional biorhythm. However, a better knowledge of your emotional cycle will help you understand why you feel as you do on certain days and why you react as you do to emotional situations.

The intellectual biorhythm

The 16½ day positive phase of your intellectual cycle is a time when you are better able to understand, absorb and retain new information. It is a time when your memory recall is at its best and when facts and figures seem to flood back with pleasing ease. Your performance in an examination or an interview would be enhanced if you could arrange these events in advance to coincide with the positive phase of your intellectual biorhythm. But, this is an option seldom open to us.

The low phase of your intellectual biorhythm is, of course, the antithesis of the positive phase. Your concentration will be impaired and you will have greater difficulty in retaining new facts or recalling stored information from your programmed memory. You may find yourself reading a passage in a book more than once in order to reach an acceptable level of understanding of the material.

We can all benefit from knowing in advance the sequence of the positive and negative phases of our intellectual biorhythm. Students, for example, should schedule more intense periods of study to coincide with the positive phase, and periods of relaxation during the negative phase. If an examination is scheduled during the negative phase it is helpful to know prior to taking the examination that your ability to recall facts may be depressed. By maintaining a relaxed state a student can still perform well, although a little more conscious effort may be involved. Students who are unaware of this phenomenon often panic and lose control over their ability to function intellectually. This is due to a need to maintain our brain waves within a certain range of excitation during memory and recall functions. Panic increases the frequency of our brain waves to a point where both programming and recall are almost negated. This is the reason people under stress are often heard to say, 'Okay, don't panic. Let's just calm down and think.'

Do individuals have different biorhythms?

The length and function of each biorhythm is exactly the same in all people and this never changes, but, the intensity of biorhythms may differ between individuals. This difference in intensity may be the reason why some individuals are more athletically inclined while others are more emotional, or perhaps given to intellectual pursuit. For example, two brothers born of the same parents may display a totally different emphasis in their biorhythmic strengths.

The older brother may be a fair student but an outstanding athlete, while the younger brother may be academically gifted but has poor physical coordination. Each brother is being driven by the intensity of his most powerful biorhythm, and perhaps limited by the correspondingly lower magnitude of his weaker biorhythms.

We can seek to maximise our efforts within the confines of the intensity of each of our biorhythms, but, there is nothing we can do to change those intensity factors. How each biorhythm presents at birth is how it will function for the remainder of our lives.

The existence of multiple biorhythmic strengths in one individual is also possible. Take for instance a person who displays a dual dominance of both the emotional and physical biorhythms. Possessing more intense emotional and physical capabilities, this person may be ideally suited to an expression such as ballet dancing. Or, a person exhibiting dual dominance of both emotional and intellectual biorhythms may best be suited to a career in psychology.

How does one biorhythm influence another?

Biorhythms are not compartmentalised and do not function independently from each other. Although one biorhythm does not directly affect the role of another, the superimposed roles of the various biorhythms will influence the way we feel and act.

For example, if your emotional biorhythm is in the positive phase you will feel positive and creative, but, if your physical biorhythm is at the bottom of the negative phase you may lack the energy to undertake certain desired tasks. Conversely, if both your emotional and your physical biorhythms were in the positive phase there may be no stopping you.

Although your biorhythms commenced simultaneous operation at the precise moment of your birth, the differing biorhythmic wave lengths will keep them apart for most of your life. Perhaps only twice in the course of your lifetime will all three meet at the apex of the positive arc and again at the apex of the negative arc. When your biorhythms meet at the apex of the positive arc you will be at your absolute best. You will be charged with physical energy, highly receptive to intellectual stimulation and have the emotional strength of a giant. If there is to be a day when you are filled with creativity and self-esteem, when you can read and understand Einstein's theory of relativity and still have the energy to dance all night, this will be the day.

Unfortunately all three of your biorhythms will also meet at the bottom of the arc of the negative phase. On these days your life will be a physical, emotional and intellectual desert.

Are some periods in a biorhythmic cycle more critical?

Yes. You are most vulnerable to accident, emotional upset or intellectual disorientation when the appropriate biorhythm is in the process of crossing the line of neutrality. As a biorhythm moves from the positive phase into the negative phase, or, from the negative phase into the positive phase you will experience a day of discord. Referred to as your critical days, these periods of transition create imbalance in the normal influence of a particular biorhythm. For example, Daniel is an active seven-year-old who likes to play on the overhead bars. He can play with reasonable control during both the positive and negative phases of his physical biorhythm, although he may tire more quickly during the bottom of his negative phase. On a physically critical day Daniel experiences an imbalance in his normal level of physical coordination and falls from the bars.

When two or even three biorhythms simultaneously cross the line of neutrality, multiple states of incoordination will prevail. A number of airlines in the United States have commissioned studies to determine the influence biorhythmic critical days are having on the ability of pilots and crew to function. In a surprising number of accidents attributed to human error, the subsequent charting of the responsible pilot's biorhythms have indicated critical days corresponding to the day of the mishap. The standing down of pilots and crew during critical days may reduce accidents and the loss of lives. Thousands of companies in Japan have initiated studies into the effects biorhythms are having on employees in such areas as manufacture, sales and decision-making. By determining each person's biorhythmic chart, industrial accidents may be reduced, better sales may result and the making of poor decisions avoided.

Can biorhythms affect relationships?

Yes, they can and they do. Your mood and your behaviour will be an extension of the influence exerted by all three biorhythms at any given moment. But, every person you contact on that day will be similarly affected by the positions of their biorhythms. Let us assume your physical biorhythm is in the positive phase and your partner's physical biorhythm is in the negative phase. On that day you will be at your physical best and your partner will be at his or her physical worst. Your heightened physical drive compels you to go on a picnic or go dancing, but your partner wants to stay at home and rest. In another 11 or 12 days when it is your partner's turn to be energetic you may well be seen as the stick-in-the-mud. Physical compatibility is best served when partners share a minimum of 65% of both good and bad days, but, the higher the percentage the more compatible will be the relationship.

The same principle applies to differences in the intellectual cycles between partners. If your intellectual biorhythms are simultaneously high you will each act to stimulate the other. If your intellectual biorhythms are in opposition you will be at your intellectual peak when your partner wants to do nothing more taxing than watch television.

Your emotional biorhythms are the exception. The positive phase of the emotional biorhythm finds us emotionally strong and seeking to give affection. The negative phase finds us emotionally vulnerable and seeking affection from others. If two people in a relationship have concurrent emotional biorhythmic highs and lows they would simultaneously alternate between periods of wanting to express emotion in the absence of a recipient, to seeking emotional support without there being a giver. Alternatively, if you are at your emotional peak when your partner is at his or her emotional ebb, you can assume the dominant role and be emotionally supportive. As your cycles change, so would your roles and your partner would become emotionally supportive of you.

Do biorhythms play any role in gaining or losing weight?

Not directly, however, indirectly your biorhythms do influence the way you feel, the rate at which you expend energy and what you eat. During the negative phase of your emotional biorhythm you may be more prone to snacking between meals. Compulsive eating is often associated with depression and low self-esteem as can be experienced with emotional biorhythmic lows. Also, compulsive eating seldom involves healthy food. As if wanting to self-punish, compulsive eaters usually consume the most fattening foods available, such as cake, cookies, chocolate and ice-cream. If this period happens to coincide with a low in a person's physical biorhythm, compulsive eating and low energy output would soon combine to form unwanted body fat.

THE 24-HOUR BIOLOGICAL CLOCK

In addition to our three major rhythms of life, our days are governed by a 24-hour biological clock. Unlike biorhythms which control our physical, emotional and intellectual cycles, our 24-hour biological clock controls the way in which we consume, process and eliminate food.

Once again, the cycle of the biological clock is of the same duration and follows the same pattern of function in all people, but, unlike biorhythms, the intensity of function does not change. Our biological day is divided into three periods each of eight hours duration (see Table 18.1).

Time period	Function	Description
noon to 8 p.m.	appropriation	ingestion and digestion of food
8 p.m. to 4 a.m.	assimilation	absorption of nutrients
4 a.m. to noon	elimination	faecal and metabolic waste disposal

The 24-hour Biological Clock
Table 18.1

The feeling of malaise associated with jet lag is partially rooted in the impact jet travel has on our 24-hour biological clock. In a bid to reduce travel boredom international airlines frequently feed their passengers. But, dinner at 3 a.m. does not sit well and the traveller usually arrives at his or her destination feeling bloated. This is due to food being appropriated and poorly digested during the elimination stage. Within a day or two the traveller's biological clock and digestive system will adjust to the new time schedule, at least until the next flight.

Essential service personnel who work a rotating roster of shifts will attest to a feeling of fullness and poor digestibility after eating meals in the wee small hours. Once again food has been consumed during the period of elimination which often leads to the onset of constipation.

Your *Slim Forever* program has been developed around the dictates of your 24-hour biological clock. By starting your day with a not-too-bulky protein breakfast you will satisfy your hunger without overloading your system. And, as protein satiates the hunger response, as opposed to carbohydrate which excites your hunger response, your perceived need to eat will be greatly reduced. At noon you will enter the appropriation period, and it is during this period the influence of your *Slim Forever* program will cause your body to mobilise fat from the fat storage cells and convert it into energy. As your body will have by now exhausted its immediate supplies of glucose from the previous evening's meal, it will look for additional carbohydrate to process into glucose. But, as you have not consumed carbohydrate for approximately 18 hours, your body will be forced to look elsewhere for its source of energy, and that source is stored body fat.

Your evening meal should not be consumed before 6 p.m. or after 8 p.m. and should include your entire daily allowance of carbohydrate. If you eat your evening meal prior to 6 p.m. you will significantly reduce the time available for losing fat as your body will quickly revert back to burning glucose for energy. If you eat too late you will suffer poor digestion, and, in the prolonged absence of dietary carbohydrate, your body may sense starvation and switch to converting muscle into glucose. By consuming your evening meal between the hours of 6 p.m. and 8 p.m. you will maximise fat loss, prevent the onset of gluconeogenesis and satisfy the appropriation demands of your 24-hour biological clock.

You should consume your evening meal a minimum of three hours before retiring to allow full digestion and expulsion of the food from your stomach. Following digestion, and for the hours remaining prior to 4 a.m., your body will absorb the nutrients from your evening meal into your bloodstream. During the elimination period commencing at 4 a.m. you will evacuate body waste and prepare for a new day of balanced eating. The carbohydrate you consumed with your evening meal will satisfy the demands of your body until around noon when you will again influence your body to burn fat for energy.

If you attempt to consume your daily allowance of carbohydrate at either breakfast or lunch you will negate the fat burning process. If your system has free access to glucose during the appropriation stage you will not lose body fat. And, as the depletion of available glucose will occur during the assimilation period, your body may revert to converting muscle into energy. Either way you will not burn body fat for energy.

As you progress with your *Slim Forever* program your body will rely less on carbohydrate and more on body fat for the production of energy, and your daily fat burning periods will lengthen. This will result in even greater losses of body fat under conditions which are absolutely safe and in keeping with the design and function of your body. For a more detailed understanding of this topic please refer to Chapter 11 *All about body fat.*

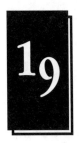

exercise, is it really necessary?

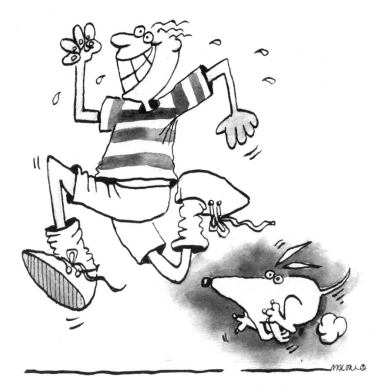

Exercise is not really necessary but it is highly desirable if you want to feel better, be healthier, and live longer. Regular daily exercise will also increase the rate at which you lose body fat. Your *Slim Forever* program will put you in the fat loss mode, but your rate of loss will be determined by how quickly you burn your excess body fat. Simply put, the more energy you use the more stored fat your body will mobilise to produce energy on each given day. But, exercise is not just about losing body fat more quickly, it is about looking good, feeling good about yourself, and living longer.

There is a down side to the positive benefits of living in a highly technological age. Apart from our apparent efforts to poison our environment and our bodies, we are compounding our health problems by becoming progressively more sedentary in our daily habits.˙ The results of a government sponsored national fitness survey released in Australia in 1992 carried some frightening revelations. Australians are justifiably proud of their country's sporting prowess, but statistically Australians are a nation of sport watchers and not sport participants. The survey indicated only 15% of the overall Australian population can be classified as being fit, with a massive 50% of the population deliberately avoiding exercise.

Physical activity among children is also on the decline, with 60% of all Australian youngsters currently classified as being either low level active or totally inactive. This unacceptable degree of inactivity has resulted in an overall lack of agility, flexibility and physical endurance in Australia's youth, and is contributing alarmingly to an underdevelopment of basic body motor skills. As a result many children enter adulthood awkward and uncoordinated.

On average, every child in the industrialised world spends four hours each day watching television or playing video games, but the adverse effects of this inactivity go beyond physical impairment. In one test children scored higher on academic exams following a period of physical activity than they did on similar exams following two hours of inactivity.

The human body functions in direct response to stimulation. The greater the magnitude of the stimulation the greater will be the function, but unfortunately the opposite also occurs. Take for example a fractured limb which has been immobilised in a plaster cast for just six to eight weeks. When the cast comes off, the limb is weak and the muscles are wasted to such an extent the patient often doubts it will ever be fully functional again. The same applies to your body. Lethargy begets lethargy, and if you don't use your muscles you will suffer a loss of body tone and function.

We can place some of the blame for our attitude towards physical exertion squarely on the shoulders of past medical science. Not too many decades ago it was generally held that exercise and sport put a strain on the heart, but the opposite is true. Sadly, people who suffered heart attacks during the first 60 years of the twentieth century were instructed to take it easy and do nothing to physically strain their ailing hearts. These already weakened hearts were compromised yet further by an imposed lifestyle often less physical than the one responsible for the problem in the first place. Not so today. Cardiac surgery patients are out of bed and exercising almost before the effects of the anaesthetic have worn off, and coronary sufferers are encouraged to exercise as a means of rehabilitation.

HOW THE BODY RESPONDS TO EXERCISE

Before we look at each of the various forms of exercise in more detail, let us first understand how and why our bodies respond as they do to physical activity. Much of the benefit from exercise has to do with the metabolic function of supplying nutrients to, and eliminating waste from, the cells of the body. The bloodstream could well be called the public transport system of the body. It is responsible for carrying oxygen, nutrients, hormones, antibodies and a host of other life-giving commodities to every one of the 75 trillion cells. This highly organised transport network systematically discharges its life supporting load as it passes by each cell, and acts as the garbage collector for carbon dioxide and metabolic waste products discharged from those same cells. Once in every full circuit of the body the blood passes through the kidneys where it deposits most of its refuse, and from there it is on to the lungs to release the carbon dioxide and pick up fresh supplies of oxygen. Then it is on to the small intestine to collect nutrients extracted from the food consumed, and the process starts all over again. The waste products extracted by the kidneys are passed off in the urine, and the carbon dioxide deposited in the lungs is expelled during exhalation.

The driving force behind this never ending flow of blood comes from the repeated contractions of a pump we call the heart. This organ is constructed of very specific muscle tissue and has no function other than to expand and contract an average of 104,000 times each day, 3,120,000 times each month or 37,960,000 each year. An enviable record for a pump so often used, abused, and never serviced during its average lifetime of more than 3,000 million contractions.

The rate at which the heart contracts is in direct response to the nutritional needs of the cells it services. High frequency exercise initiates an increase in cellular activity which in turn places greater demand on the supply of glucose, triglycerides, oxygen and other nutrients from the bloodstream. The body accommodates this increase in demand by moving the blood more quickly through the body, and to some extent by increasing the concentrations of some of the blood borne nutrients. But, it is speed of transport rather than increased concentrations of nutrients that fulfils most of the additional demand. Any increase in the need for oxygen and nutrients gives rise to an increase in overall heart rate, and the heart gets to exercise by default. Like the muscles in your arms or legs or around your waist, the muscle of your heart will respond positively to exercise and will become stronger, display better tone and will last longer. Conversely, the heart will become weak and soft if it is not regularly stimulated by exercise.

GETTING FIT

If you have not exercised for some time, or if you have never really exercised, it will take a little time before you start to get fit. Getting fit really means your body is reacting to the demands placed upon it to perform physical exercise. As the intensity of the exercise increases your muscles will proportionately increase in tone, strength and energy producing capacity. Detailed information on how muscles react to the stimulus of exercise is presented in Chapter 20 *Building muscle*.

Regular exercise will increase your ability to produce energy, but the benefits you will enjoy will go beyond the time you spend exercising. Each muscle cell under load will manufacture mitochondria in sufficient quantities to produce the energy necessary to accommodate your current exercise routine. Therefore, the more you exercise the greater will be your capacity to produce energy. Getting fit involves exercising at a level compatible with your current ability to produce energy, and then progressively increasing the intensity of your routine to force your body to produce even more energy. Within weeks you will reach an acceptable level of fitness and energy production, but your body will retain the capacity to produce that same level of energy even when you are not exercising. The hours of the day not devoted to exercise will be filled with a vibrant desire to get up and go and to be involved – and isn't that what life is all about?

Some helpful hints

The following suggestions will be of help in getting you started on a regular exercise program.

- Do not set yourself an impossible exercise routine. If you aim too high in the beginning you will quickly become disillusioned and probably quit.

- Learn as much as you can about the exercise routine you are about to follow. Exercising is an art and should be treated accordingly to prevent injury.

- Ease into your program and give your body time to respond. If you extend yourself too quickly and overtax your muscles you will be made to suffer the consequences, at least for a few days.

- Climb your exercise ladder a rung at a time. You will achieve your desired level of fitness if you constantly and progressively challenge your current physical barrier, not by mounting an all out assault.

■ Make exercise part of your daily routine but don't get into the habit of contemplating your next workout. It is easy to talk yourself out of exercising if you dwell on what you are about to do.

Apathy and lethargy are the sworn enemies of physical fitness. Most of us go to work because we have to, but we often forego our obligation to exercise simply because we are not sufficiently motivated. We make excuses for the things we don't feel compelled to undertake, and exercise is no exception. A little exercise every day is much like putting money in the bank — you get it back with interest when you need it most. But, more importantly you will feel better within yourself, and about yourself, every single day for the rest of your life. There is nothing you can do to change your life up to this moment, but there is certainly lots you can do to change your life from this moment on. Remember, today is the first day of the rest of your life, so make the most of it.

Too old? Never! We age prematurely because we allow our bodies to waste away through lack of use. Everyone can, and will, benefit from exercise, and remember, you don't have to be an athlete to participate. Include exercise in your daily routine, follow a sensible program you can live with and the short and long-term results will amaze you. Life is for living, but you have to be fully alive to reap the benefits.

STRETCHING BEFORE EXERCISING

An animal will seldom move away from the sitting or lying position without stretching. Most children instinctively stretch when they awaken, but adults seldom do. A muscle not fully stretched is prone to injury, so whatever your chosen sport or exercise routine, take a few minutes to stretch out before you commence. Stretching will not only drastically reduce the probability of injury, it will make you perform better.

Here are a number of stretching exercises you may find helpful.

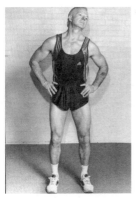

◀ Neck Rolling

Stand with feet comfortably apart and with hands on hips, bend your neck to the side and try to touch your right ear to your right shoulder. Now roll your head back, around to the left, then forward and back again to your starting position. Alternate by touching your left ear to your left shoulder and rotating your head in a counter-clockwise direction. Perform three rotations in each direction.

Trunk rotations ▶▶

Maintain your standing position with feet comfortably apart and arms extended out from your body. Rotate your trunk to the left extending your outstretched arms as far back as you can comfortably reach. Return to the starting position and repeat the exercise to the right. Perform three times in each direction.

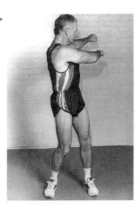

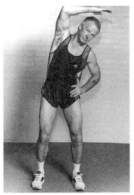

◀ Lateral trunk extensions

In the standing position with your feet comfortably apart, place your left hand on your left hip and raise your right arm above your head. Bend your torso to the left and extend your outstretched right arm as far as you can to the left. Return to the standing position and repeat the exercise with your right hand on your right hip and your left arm extended upwards, extending to the right. Perform the exercise three times in each direction.

Trunk flexion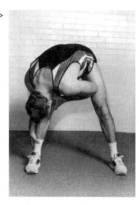

Stand with your feet approximately shoulder width apart. Bend forward and grasp the right ankle with your right hand, and with your left hand on your right knee, pull your upper body down and attempt to touch your right knee with your forehead. Move your left hand to your left ankle and your right hand to your left knee and repeat the procedure. Perform the exercise three times each side.

◀ Stretching the thigh muscles

Support yourself against a wall or fence with your left hand. Raise your right heel to your buttocks, grasping your ankle with your right hand. Pull your foot upwards, stretching the quadriceps muscles in the front of the thigh. Lower your leg and repeat the exercise by grasping your left ankle with your left hand. Perform three times with each leg.

Stretching the hamstrings and ▶ muscles of the buttocks

Stand with your back pressed against a wall with your heels positioned approximately 1 ft/300 mm out from the wall. Take your weight on one leg and raise the other leg, flexing it at the knee. Reach out with both arms and grasp the knee, drawing it up to your chest. Lower the leg and alternately perform the exercise three times with each leg.

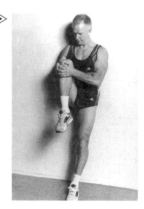

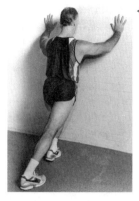

◄ Stretching the calf muscles

Stand at a distance approximately equal to your height from a wall or fence. Lean forward with arms outstretched and support yourself against the wall or fence. Bring the left leg forward, keeping your weight on your outstretched right leg. Force downwards on your right heel stretching the calf muscle. Change legs and repeat the exercise three times for each calf muscle.

When we are in a relaxed state only the belly or middle portion of the muscle is used. A relaxed muscle which is required to quickly extend to its full length under load, without first having been stretched, will often become strained. Protect your body by stretching at least once each day. Perform the exercises slowly and to the full extent of muscle extension, holding the stretch for a few seconds.

TYPES OF EXERCISE

Exercise falls into two distinct categories, the first of which is cardiovascular. This is an exercise regimen designed specifically to strengthen the muscles of the heart and to expand and contract the arteries. These actions combine to increase the magnitude of the blood flow to and from every nook and cranny in your body. The second category is isotonic exercise specifically designed to extend, contract and strengthen the skeletal muscles, with or without resistance of additional weight.

Isotonic exercise usually involves a degree of cardiovascular exercise, and cardiovascular exercise embraces a degree of isotonic exercise. However, few exercise routines, with the possible exception of properly choreographed aerobics, place sufficient emphasis on both types of activity. If you have to make a choice between the two, choose cardiovascular, but ideally you should perform both cardiovascular and isotonic exercises on a daily basis.

Let us now look at some of the various exercise options.

Jogging

Jogging is perhaps the best of all the cardiovascular exercises. Excellent cardiovascular function can be achieved by increasing the heart rate to above 140 beats per minute by jogging, and maintaining that rate for a minimum of 26 minutes at least three times each week. There are 168 hours in every week and for just $1\frac{1}{2}$ of those hours spent jogging, every person alive could maintain a level of cardiovascular fitness capable of eliminating heart disease as a major cause of death in our society.

To run is a natural extension of the design of the human body, and run our forebears did if they wanted to eat. Children are blessed with the inherent ability to run, and they do so with grace and fluid motion, but the instinctive ability is soon lost in adulthood due to practised inactivity. Adults who have not broken into a trot since childhood appear awkward and uncoordinated, but the lost art of running can be recaptured with a little effort and fortitude.

As with every field of endeavour, too many people with too little knowledge have had something to say about jogging, much of which is untrue. If our ankles, knees, hips and kidneys were not designed to withstand the rigours of running we would not have developed the ability to run in the first place. However, our environment has changed considerably during the years of industrialisation and the urban jogger of today is confronted with more asphalt and concrete than wide open spaces. If you have a choice, select a softer surface as jogging on a hard surface can cause injury if not performed correctly. If either asphalt or concrete is your only alternative you can run without injury provided you adhere to the following suggestions.

The necessary equipment

Jogging is possibly the most physically rewarding and the least expensive of all the cardiovascular exercises, and it is not too bulky to take on business trips or on vacation. To get the most from your time spent jogging, and to prevent any possible injury, purchase a good set of jogging shoes. Modern technology has produced running shoes which are superb to wear, light in weight and often with air bag heels which are designed to eliminate almost all ground shock. Choose a good pair of well fitting jogging shoes and don't be too cheap with your purchase – they will last for years.

Jogging demands you dress with light, loose clothing to allow air to reach the pores of your skin. The less clothing you wear the better you will perform, and under no circumstances go jogging wearing rubberised or plastic pants or tops. Contrary to popular belief, it is impossible to lose body fat by perspiring. Plastic and rubber clothing will only serve to suffocate your skin, and you will run the risk of serious overheating. Wear a cotton track suit in cold weather, and natural cotton socks, and above all, wear a good pair of jogging shoes.

Properly dressed and fully stretched, it is now time to go for a run. If this is a relatively new experience for you, the following suggestions may be of assistance in getting you started.

■ *Do not jog with your hands above your waist*
Jog with your hands lightly clenched and below the level of your waist. Clenched fists and a pumping action with your arms bent will restrict the expanding action of your rib cage and impair your breathing. The secret to performing any exercise well is to be relaxed at all times, so don't tense any muscles unnecessarily. A muscle under constant contraction will use a lot of precious energy and your body and your muscles will quickly fatigue.

■ *Run across the ground, not into it*
If you can hear your feet slapping you are running into the ground, and not over the top of it. Project yourself forward across the running surface and concentrate on caressing the ground with your feet, not compressing it.

■ *Breathe though your nose and your mouth*
Nasal breathing when jogging will seriously restrict the flow of air to your lungs. A jogging body needs lots of oxygen so breathe deeply through the mouth and nose at the same time. Air is one of the few things left that is free, so gulp it down.

■ *Use your diaphragm fully*
Correct breathing is perhaps the most important part of any physical endeavour. Unfortunately, many of us have been raised to pull our stomach in, push our chest out, tuck our chin in and look up. This restrictive posture is the cause of many soldiers collapsing on the parade ground due to partial asphyxiation. They simply don't get enough air into their lungs. During inhalation, the rib cage expands outwards and the diaphragm contracts downwards into the abdomen allowing the air to rush in. Don't do anything to restrict these actions.

■ *Jog from the waist down*
It is important you remain relaxed while you are jogging by involving your trunk, arms, head and neck as little as possible. Concentrate on running from the waist down and in time you will develop an easy rolling and totally relaxed motion of the hips.

■ *Lean forward when running uphill*
Running up an incline becomes easier if you lean forward and reach out with your loosely clawed hands. With palms turned downward, reach out with each hand in turn and imagine you are pulling yourself up the hill – it really works.

■ *Jog for time, not for speed or distance*
Set yourself a goal of time rather than distance or speed. You should jog for at least 26 minutes and your run should be completed within your current physical capabilities. Commence by alternating walking with jogging. As your physical fitness improves, reduce the frequency and the duration of walking and increase your jogging until you can complete your allotted time without walking at all. During this build-up period try to perform a little better each day. Many of us give up too easily, so try running until you feel you can't possibly run another step, then run 20 more paces before you commence your next walking period. As your physical condition

improves so too will your speed and the distance you cover. Give yourself time to improve, and remember the only race you are training for is a place in the human race. Sensible exercise wins hands down every time.

Walking

Fast walking became popular when much was being said to the detriment of jogging. Walking is a good exercise but it must be classified as a soft cardiovascular exercise. While it is an improvement over a stroll in the park, the cardiovascular gain is less than you will experience with jogging.

Many fast walkers attempt to combine walking with isotonic exercise by clenching their fists, bending their elbows and pumping their arms and shoulders. Some even carry mini dumbbells. The rules for running apply to walking, and the upper trunk should be left as relaxed as possible to avoid restriction of breathing. Wear light clothing and a good pair of running shoes, and remember the faster you walk the greater will be your cardiovascular rewards. Above all, perform your skeletal muscle exercise either before or after your walk, not during it.

Bicycle riding

There is a trend back to riding bicycles, but a gentle peddle around the park is a little like taking a stroll while sitting down. Bicycle riding with the challenge of distance and a few hills provides good cardiovascular exercise with the added benefit of exercising the leg muscles, and to a lesser degree the muscles of the abdomen and low back. Venue may be a problem if you are an urban dweller. Finding a stretch of road or track free from the threat of injury associated with vehicular traffic and toxic exhaust fumes is sometimes difficult.

Stretch before you start riding and carry drinking water with you on hot days to prevent dehydration. As with any exercise routine, start slowly and steadily increase your speed and the distance you travel to coincide with your improving physical condition.

Aerobics

Most work-outs are specifically choreographed to be of low impact and devoid of any jarring movements. Aerobics is perhaps the only exercise routine offering an acceptable combination of both cardiovascular and isotonic exercise. The cardiovascular component may not be as good as jogging, and the isotonic portion may not be as effective as working with weights, but it is still an excellent form of exercise.

The level of physical involvement of an aerobics program is usually tailored to complement the physical condition of the participant. Programs are offered ranging from those developed for beginners, to programs which are totally exhausting. Aerobics can be undertaken in the privacy of your own home following your own program or a prerecorded program on video, or in organised classes which do have much to offer. Organised classes have the added advantages of changes in routine to avoid boredom, peer support and professional guidance. It should not be too difficult to fit an aerobics work-out into your busy schedule as the majority of commercial health clubs offer classes at various times of the day and evening. If your desire is to reach and maintain an acceptable level of cardiovascular and muscle fitness, and you feel you would benefit from being in a committed class environment, a health club may well be your ticket.

Good general purpose athletic shoes are relatively inexpensive and an old pair of shorts and a shirt will do, but you can spend a lot of money on designer work-out gear if you wish. Where practical, women should wear an athletic bra for support when performing any sporting activity, especially when jogging or performing an aerobics routine.

Swimming

Regular swimming sessions offer a good form of exercise with reasonable cardiovascular and isotonic benefits, although many athletes train in a gymnasium to increase their in-water strength. Swimming is an excellent choice of exercise for the injured, the aged and the infirmed as the swimmer's body is largely supported by water and not subjected to jarring or shock.

Unless a pool is heated, swimming year round in most climates can be difficult. If you choose swimming you may need to consider an alternative exercise routine for the cooler months. If you are a novice and you are contemplating swimming as an exercise you should seek the expert advice of the pool coach before you commence.

Body building

Body building is isotonic exercise against resistance. As with any physical endeavour, exercising to improve your body is an art and all art must be learned. To learn the art of body building the newcomer should seek the expert guidance of trained health club staff and watch the training procedures of other more experienced body builders. A vast array of magazines on the subject of body building also present articles on training techniques.

Perhaps our greatest collective human failing is our inability as individuals to accept ourselves for who and what we really are. This philosophy also applies to body building, so seek to maximise your natural muscularity and avoid over development. Unnaturally large muscles are redundant to any other activity other than lifting heavy weights, so what is the point in carrying extra poundage around with you if it is of no benefit in your daily life? Seek to develop a body complementary to your genetic physical structure and do it for the benefit of your personal health and well-being, not to impress others. For more detailed information regarding safe and healthy muscle development please refer to Chapter 20 *Building muscle.*

Other forms of exercise

There are many forms of exercise not mentioned here. Tai chi, martial arts, tennis, squash, racquet ball, hockey, basketball, football and many of the other more active sporting activities are all commendable forms of exercise provided the activity is performed regularly. A once a week game of any sport will not be sufficient physical stimulation if you are seeking to develop optimum physical well-being. But, if your occasional game is performed in conjunction with other cardiovascular and isotonic exercises your performance on and off the playing field will no doubt improve.

Regular exercise will improve your life in so many ways. You will sleep, think, work and play better and you will be a happier and a more contented person. Diminished sexual drive due to high stress living and poor physical well-being is the cause of many failed relationships. Exercise, like alcohol, is a stimulant. However, unlike alcohol which increases the desire but often inhibits the performance, regular exercise increases both the desire and the performance. Maybe regular exercise isn't such a bad idea after all!

2_0 *building muscle*

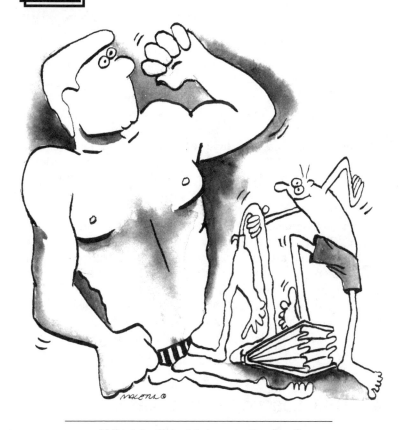

What builds bigger muscles?

Why do muscle cells increase in size?

What type of exercise builds muscles?

Muscle building food

Fat off, muscle on

Building bigger and stronger muscles is not a subject of interest to everyone. But, there is an undeniable portion of the world population who would like to be more muscular if only they knew how to achieve their purpose. Desire for increased muscularity aside, the average person in the western world suffers muscular underdevelopment. Not so much in size but in muscle density and tone.

We tend to think of muscles as being the bits that bulge in our arms and legs, but we have muscles everywhere performing all manner of functions. Our blood is kept in perpetual motion by the pumping action of the heart, an organ made almost entirely of muscle. The initial propulsive force applied to the blood by the heart is augmented by tiny contractions of bands of muscle in the walls of the arteries. In a similar fashion, food in the digestive tract is propelled forward by the rhythmic contractions of tiny muscles in the wall of the intestine. The movement of fluids within the body and the retention and release of body excretions are controlled by a highly organised system of muscular valves. Frowning, smiling, eating, blinking, waving, kicking and even hair standing on end are all examples of highly integrated muscle systems in action. However, the efficiency of a muscle to function is governed by the degree of fitness of that muscle. This is referred to as muscle tone.

We tend to identify more readily with our skeletal muscle groups such as those in our arms, legs and back, simply because they are more visually apparent to us. But, if the muscles we can see are weak, it is highly probable the ones we cannot see are also weak.

WHAT BUILDS BIGGER MUSCLES?

Muscle strength and growth are dependent upon two regulatory factors, dietary protein and exercise. If a muscle is to become fully developed a person must consume sufficient protein on a daily basis to effect optimum tissue reconstruction. However, muscles are lazy and will only fully develop if they are subjected to regular load bearing exercise.

Provided our bodies remain anatomically intact, we will retain the same number of muscle cells throughout our entire lives. Pee Wee Herman and Arnold Schwarzenegger have very different physiques, but, despite their differences in muscular development they each have exactly the same number of muscle cells. In Arnold's case the contents of his muscle cells are greatly increased, contributing to his increase in muscularity.

WHY DO MUSCLE CELLS INCREASE IN SIZE?

A muscle cell is a little like an inflated balloon with the surface of the balloon representing the cell wall. This wall forms a selective barrier between the nutrient-rich blood on the outside and a liquid substance on the inside of the cell called cytoplasm. In the middle of the cell is another tiny balloon-like structure called a nucleus which contains the reproductive and control apparatus. Floating around in the gel-like cytoplasm is a network of working parts called organelles with exotic names such as mitochondria, endoplasmic reticula and golgi complexes. The organelles of specific interest to us in the context of building muscle are the mitochondria.

What are mitochondria?

Mitochondria can best be described as the powerhouses of the muscle cells. Their function is to absorb nutrients from the cytoplasm and convert these nutrients into a substance called adenosine triphosphate (ATP). ATP is generated principally from glucose and fats and supplies the energy necessary for muscle contraction.

Mitochondria are self-replicating. That is to say, each mitochondrion is capable of forming a multiplicity of new mitochondria. The number of mitochondria a cell contains is directly proportional to the energy demands placed on the body. Muscle cells with little demand for work may contain only a few hundred mitochondria, but, a very active cell can contain many thousands. It is the sum of the mitochondria in the cells of a muscle and the enlargement of the muscle fibres that determine the overall size, strength and endurance of the muscle itself.

To increase muscle size you must first challenge your muscles to work harder, and this can only be by undertaking a program of resistance exercise. But, you cannot take a muscle containing relatively few mitochondria and bludgeon them into producing more energy. The energy producing potential of each mitochondrion is very specific, and nothing you do will induce an increase in production above that potential. Additional energy can only be generated by increasing the number of mitochondria a cell contains. If you have been leading a sedentary lifestyle the number of mitochondria in your muscle cells will probably be on the low end of the scale. A low mitochondrial count means reduced energy potential which will in turn limit the amount of exercise you can perform before reaching exhaustion.

How to get more mitochondria

As each mitochondrion has a limited potential to produce energy, your body will respond to any increase in energy demand by producing more of these little powerhouses. Commence exercising within your present energy producing capabilities and consistently increase the intensity of your exercise routine over time. Your body will respond by producing more mitochondria, but they will not suddenly appear overnight. It is for this reason the first two or three weeks of exercising will be your most difficult. It is also during this period when most people quit, so be persistent. Your persistence will be rewarded with an increase in available energy and you will be on your way to getting fit.

You can relate the process of getting fit to climbing a flight of stairs. The further you go up the stairs the fitter you will become, and, with persistence, you will reach the top. This concept was exemplified in the movie *Rocky* when Sylvester Stallone finally made it to the top of the steps at City Hall. He danced with his arms stretched above his head in a V for victory sign signifying he had successfully broken through the energy barrier.

Unfortunately, the process of producing mitochondria by increasing your need for energy can also work in reverse. If at any time you find yourself back at the bottom of the stairs, the number of mitochondria within your muscles will decrease accordingly. As the intensity of your exercise program diminishes, so too will your energy, your endurance and your strength. But, on a more positive note there is a wonderful spin-off from exercising. Your increased capacity to produce energy sufficient to get you through the most arduous part of your exercise routine will stay with you 24 hours a day. Your muscles will quickly recover from your work-out and you will be free to enjoy an abundance of energy perhaps not previously experienced.

WHAT TYPE OF EXERCISE BUILDS MUSCLES?

Your muscles will grow in proportion to the level of load bearing exercise you perform. If you walk, jog or undertake regular aerobics you will achieve better muscle tone and you may even increase the size of the muscles you are using. But, as always, there is a limit. You will eventually reach a point of energy production and muscle tone commensurate with the level of intensity of the exercise you perform. For example, if you were to undertake 45 minutes of aerobics every day you would reach a level of muscular development equal to the demands of that particular exercise routine. However, by increasing your aerobics routine to 90 minutes you may not significantly increase your muscular development. This is because the intensity of your routine will not have increased, just the duration.

If you seek appreciable muscular development you will need to undertake load bearing exercises using progressively heavier resistance. This can only be achieved by exercising with weights.

How hard and how often to exercise

Your level of increased muscular development will depend upon the amount of exercise you undertake both in terms of intensity and duration, but there are limits. Although many competitive body builders exercise for hours each day, you can achieve excellent results with much shorter work-out periods.

You will gain from exercise what you put into it. If you only seek a level of pleasing muscle tone with increased vitality, you can achieve your goal with three exercise periods of between 40 and 60 minutes each week. If your desire is to maximise muscle development you will have to consider five or six exercise sessions each week.

What makes a good exercise routine?

Body building magazines are full of articles depicting specific exercise routines favoured by reigning and budding champions. There are almost as many routines as there are body builders, but to be effective an exercise format should embrace the following criteria:

- an exercise routine should be performed on a regular basis;

- the exercises performed during each session should concentrate on a specific group of muscles;

- emphasis should be placed on performing each exercise correctly and not on the weight being used;

- each exercise should be performed to the extremes of muscle contraction and extension and be sufficiently repetitious to fully work the muscle; and

- coincide the intensity of your exercise program with your 23-day physical biorhythm cycle.

Regularity of performance

If you choose to exercise three days each week you should do so with at least one day of no exercise in between. For example, exercising on Monday, Wednesday and Friday will be more beneficial than training on say Monday, Tuesday and Wednesday. If you choose a four day routine, group your routine into two lots of two consecutive days with a one and a two day rest in between. A five day routine can be performed on five consecutive days with a two day rest period, or you could choose a two and a three day period with just one day in between each exercise period. A six day routine gives you no choice other than to take every seventh day as a rest day.

If you don't mind when your rest days fall you may choose to work out on alternate days, or for two or three consecutive days with one rest day in between.

Muscle grouping of exercises

When a muscle is under physical load your body will fill the tissue in that area with oxygen and nutrient enriched blood. Body builders refer to this as 'pumping a muscle'. Without the benefit of oxygen and nutrients your muscles would soon fatigue and growth would be impossible. If you constantly switch between muscle groups your body will not have time to concentrate blood into each of those areas, and growth will suffer.

You will obtain your best possible results by dividing your body into anatomical areas. For three and six day routine you may choose the following routine:

- day 1 – chest and biceps
- day 2 – back and shoulders
- day 3 – legs and triceps.

The legs and the triceps may seem too far apart to be effectively exercised in the same session, but this is the exception. The triceps are a relatively small muscle group and do not require a lot of blood under load. If your exercise routine is structured to concentrate initially on the legs and then to incorporate triceps exercises, the transition will be totally effective.

If your exercise routine is on a three day schedule you will exercise each muscle group once during the course of each week. If you may choose a six day routine and you will perform each exercise routine twice during the course of each week. If your routine calls for five days of exercise you will exercise some muscle groups twice and others only once. But, by simply starting each new week where you left off at the end of the previous week you will exercise each body part equally over time.

If you schedule four exercise sessions each week you can adopt the same ongoing routine as for five exercise sessions. Or, you may decided you want to work all of your body twice during the course of each week as follows:

- day 1 – chest, back and shoulders
- day 2 – legs, biceps and triceps.

Learning the art

There is an art to training with weights, an art you must seek to acquire. Any exercise involving the resistance of weight which is performed incorrectly will expose you to injury and rob you of the positive results you seek. The following hints may be of benefit to you.

- If an exercise requires you to stand, do so with your feet comfortably apart at a distance of approximately 75% of your shoulder width. Standing with feet together reduces the support of the lower abdominal muscles and herniation could occur.

- When lifting weights from the floor arch your back forward, look up and bend your knees.

- When exercising your upper body in the supine position (lying on your back) place your feet squarely on the floor, arch your back slightly forward and press your shoulder blades into the bench.

- Make sure you are balanced and comfortable before you lift a weight. Imbalance is a major cause of injury when exercising with weights.

- Under no circumstances should you rotate your trunk when your body is under load. Twisting will disengage the erector muscles of the low back and exert a shearing action on the vertebrae and discs of the lumbar spine.

- Breathe correctly. Gulp air in through your mouth and nose to fill your lungs with oxygen. Your body will be producing lots of carbon dioxide during exercise so blast the air out and clear your lungs before you inhale.

- Keep your mind on what you are doing and focus your mental attention on the muscle group you are exercising. If your body is in the gymnasium but your mind is elsewhere, you may as well go and join it.

- Take note of the style exhibited by experienced body builders and learn from their experience.

Learning the language

For newcomers to weight training, the term *set* refers to a single exercise routine. Each set requires you to perform the exercise a number of times and these are referred to as *repetitions* or *reps*. For example, if your exercise routine requires 4 sets of 12 repetitions you would perform the exercise 12 times, rest, and repeat the procedure until all 4 sets have been completed.

Other words you will encounter will include *pump* which means filling a muscle with blood by exercise, and *burn* which describes the feeling associated with a muscle under extreme load. Word shortening is also a favourite of body builders when referring to specific muscles. For example, *abs* refers to the abdominal muscles, *pecs* to the pectorals on the front of the chest, and *lats* to the latissimus dorsi muscles under the arms and across the back. The word *traps* refers to the trapezius muscles running from the top of your shoulder to the neck, and *gluts* to the gluteal muscles of the buttocks. In the legs there are the *hammies* which refer to the hamstring group of muscles at the back of the thigh, and *quads* meaning the quadriceps group at the front of the thigh.

Exercising all of a muscle

The quest for lifting heavy weights often results in exercising only the middle part or 'belly' of a muscle. This can be avoided if you:

- ■ Choose a weight you can handle without placing overdue strain on your body. If you are performing 4 sets of 12 reps your choice of weight should allow you to complete all 12 reps in the first 2 sets, at least 10 reps in the third set and 8 in the final set. When you can comfortably complete all 4 sets of 12 reps increase the weight slightly and repeat the process.

- ■ Do not throw the weight to get it mobile or allow the weight to drop during the return phase of an exercise. You only achieve results when you maintain even pressure on a muscle during both the flexion and extension phases of an exercise.

- ■ Exercise each muscle from full flexion to full extension. If you exercise using a short jerking motion you will restrict load to the middle portion of the muscle and it will become chunky and lack symmetry.

Using your physical biorhythm to advantage

Constantly exercising at the same level of intensity will be tiring and you may become bored and give up. You should plan your exercise program to constantly rise to a peak of performance and then reduce slightly in intensity. Each time you extend yourself your performance should improve over your previous peak. This you can do only if your body has had time to recover.

You will achieve your best results if you take advantage of the influence of your physical biorhythmic cycle. Please refer to Chapter 19 *Biorhythms and biological clocks* for a better understanding of biorhythms and how they influence our lives and our bodies. Your performance will improve dramatically during the positive cycle of your physical biorhythm and this should be the focus of your greatest effort.

You may have your biorhythms charted by one of the many individuals or firms offering this service, or you can take note of your performance and mark on a calendar the day your energy level is at its lowest ebb. This will be the bottom of the negative phase of your physical biorhythm and a good starting point for future calculations.

One complete cycle of your physical biorhythm occupies a period of 23 days, but in reality you will have approximately 12 days of good performance, six days of medium performance and five days of poor performance (see Figure 20.1).

The poor performance period of your physical biorhythm should be used to recuperate and reactivate your level of energy. If you wish to take a short break from your exercise routine this will be the ideal time. However, if you are committed to continuing without a break you should reduce your peak performance weights by at least 20%. You may also consider reducing the number of sets you perform during this period. If you rest or reduce your exercise load during your poor physical days your body will perform better in the weeks to come.

As you enter the first period of medium performance you should gradually increase your weights and your physical activity. Once in the positive cycle you can pull out all the stops and aim to coincide your best effort with the peak of your physical

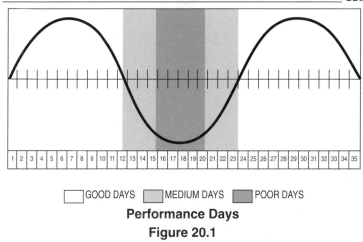

GOOD DAYS MEDIUM DAYS POOR DAYS

Performance Days

Figure 20.1

biorhythm. Reduce the intensity of your routine and the weights you are using during the second medium performance period and prepare to rest again during the recuperation phase.

In practice you will not have to watch the calendar to know where you are on your physical cycle. Once you become aware of the effects of the physical biorhythm your body will tell you when to increase and when to reduce the intensity of your routine, provided you listen. Many body builders try to overcome the feeling of lethargy by working even harder, but the results are seldom positive. Their lack of physical ability is aggravated by frustration and they enter their most productive exercise period tired and unable to achieve optimum results.

A routine to try

The author has been exercising with weights for 36 years and has developed the following exercise routine. You may wish to vary the exercises or the sequence to suit your purpose, but it will give you somewhere to start.

This exercise program was developed using the principle of *super-setting.* This means alternating between two complementary exercises each focusing on slightly different muscles. If you perform each exercise singularly you will spend a large portion of your work-out period resting. But, by slightly altering the focus of exercise you can alternate from one exercise to the other and have less rest in between. Super-setting keeps the area you are exercising pumped with blood, increases your overall level of fitness and reduces the time you spend in the gymnasium.

The exercises are presented in pairs and demonstrated in photographic form. You should super-set each pair of exercises in the order they are presented. The term *supine* means lying on your back, and the term *prone* means lying face down. *Flexion* refers to any movement toward your body, and *extension* to any movement away from your body. To better understand the concept of flexion and extension try these very simple exercises. Clench your hands, press your toes downward and curl up into the foetal position. Every movement of every joint and muscle will then be in a state of flexion. Now, if you jump into the air with arms, legs, fingers, toes and head outstretched, your body will be in total extension.

The following program is suitable for both females and males.

THREE DAY EXERCISE PROGRAM

Day 1 - Chest and biceps

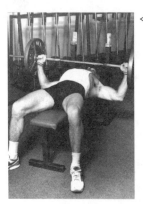

◀ **Bench press**
Muscle group – pectorals
Position – supine
Breathe – in on flexion
Sets – 4 by 12

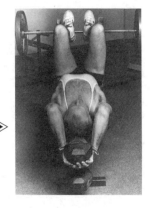

Dumbbell pull-overs   ▶▶
Muscle group – pectorals
Position – supine
Breathe – in on extension
Sets – 4 by 12

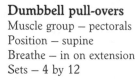

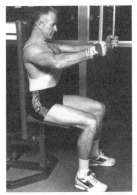

◀ Flying machine
Muscle group – pectorals
Position – sitting
Breathe – in on extension
Sets – 4 by 12

Bent bar preacher curls
Muscle group – biceps
Position – sitting
Breathe – in on flexion
Sets – 4 by 12

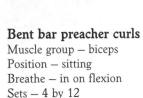

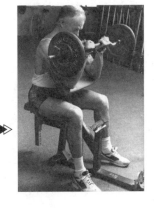

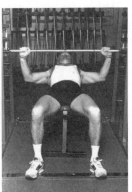

◀ Inclined bench press
Muscle group – pectorals
Position – sitting
Breathe – in on flexion
Sets – 4 by 12

Dumbbell curls
Muscle group – biceps
Position – standing
Breathe – in on flexion
Sets – 4 by 12

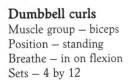

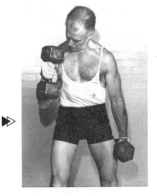

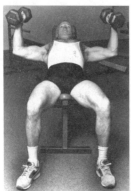

◀ Inclined flying
Muscle group – pectorals
Position – supine
Breathe – in on extension
Sets – 4 by 12

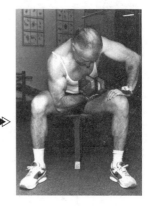

Restricted dumbbell curls ▶▶
Muscle group – biceps
Position – sitting
Breathe – in on flexion
Sets – 4 by 12

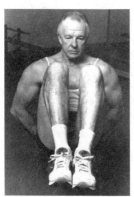

◀ Sit-ups with leg flexion
Muscle group – abdominal
Position – supine
Breathe – in on flexion
Sets – 4 by 20 plus

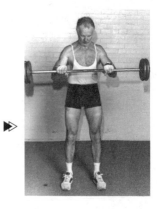

Reverse barbell curls ▶▶
Muscle group – forearms
Position – standing
Breathe – in on flexion
Sets – 4 by 12

Day 2 - Back and shoulders

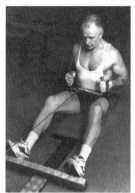

◀◀Rowing machine
Muscle group – upper back
Position – sitting
Breathe – in on flexion
Sets – 4 by 12

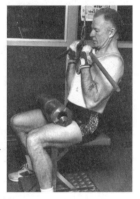

Narrow grip pull-downs to chest ▶▶
Muscle group – latissimus dorsi
Position – sitting
Breathe – in on flexion
Sets – 4 by 12

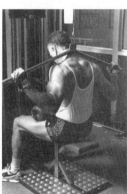

◀◀Wide grip pull-downs to neck
Muscle group – lattissimus dorsi
Position – sitting
Breathe – in on flexion
Sets – 4 by 12

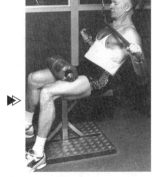

Wide grip pull-downs to chest ▶▶
Muscle group – latissimus dorsi
Position – sitting
Breathe – in on flexion
Sets – 4 by 12

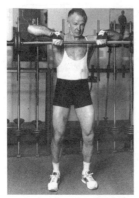

◀ Upright rowing
Muscle group – deltoids and trapezius
Position – standing
Breathe – in on flexion
Sets – 4 by 12

Bent-over dumbbell rowing 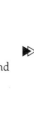
Muscle group – supraspinatus and
                 rhomboids
Position – standing
Breathe – in on flexion
Sets – 4 by 12

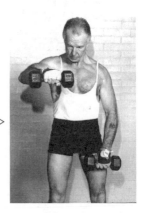

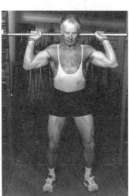

◀ Military press to neck
Muscle group – deltoids and trapezius
Position – standing
Breathe – in on flexion
Sets – 4 by 12

Forward dumbbell extensions   ▶▶
Muscle group – deltoids and trapezius
Position – standing
Breathe – in on extension
Sets – 4 by 12

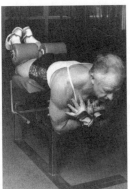

◀◀ Lumbar extensions

Muscle group – erector spinae
Position – prone
Breathe – in on extension
Sets – 4 by 20 plus

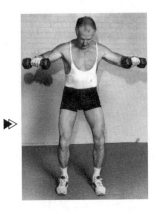

Lateral dumbbell extensions ▶▶

Muscle group – deltoids and
                        trapezius
Position – standing
Breathe – in on extension
Sets – 4 by 12

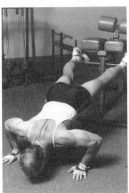

◀◀ Body presses

Muscle group – supraspinatus and rhomboids
Position – prone
Breathe – in on flexion
Sets – 4 by 20 plus

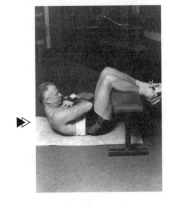

Abdominal crunches ▶▶

Muscle group – abdominal
Position – supine
Breathe – in on extension
Sets – 4 by 20 plus

Day 3 - Legs and triceps

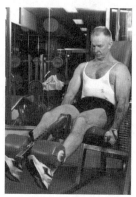

◀ Leg extensions
Muscle group – quadriceps
Position – sitting
Breathe – in on extension
Sets – 4 by
15

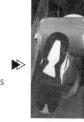

Leg curls
Muscle group – hamstrings and gluteals
Position – prone
Breathe – in on flexion
Sets – 4 by 15

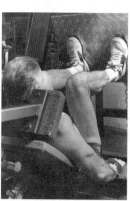

◀ Leg press
Muscle group – quadriceps and gluteals
Position – sitting
Breathe – in on flexion
Sets – 4 by 15

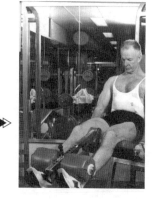

Triceps dips
Muscle group – triceps
Position – suspended
Breathe – in on flexion
Sets – 4 by 12

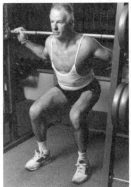

◀ Squats
Muscle group – quadriceps and gluteals
Position – standing
Breathe – in on flexion
Sets – 4 by 15

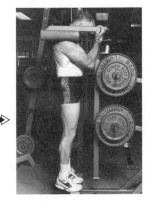

Calves   ▷▷
Muscle group – gastrocnemius and
             soleus
Position – standing
Breathe – in on flexion
Sets – 4 by 20

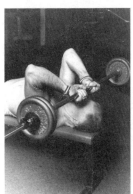

◀ Barbell tricpes curls
Muscle group – triceps
Position – supine
Breathe – in on flexion
Sets – 4 by 12

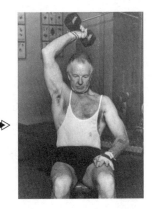

Dumbbell triceps curls   ▷▷
Muscle group – triceps
Position – sitting
Breathe – in on flexion
Sets – 4 by 12

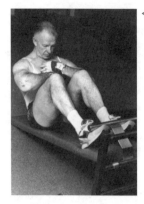

◀ Declined sit-ups
Muscle group – abdominal
Position – supine
Breathe – in on extension
Sets – 4 by 20 plus

Triceps extensions
Muscle group – triceps
Position – standing
Breathe – in on extension
Sets – 4 by 12

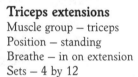

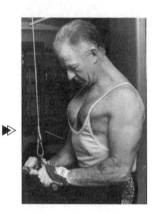

How much muscle is enough

The building of muscle out of all proportion to the performance of daily tasks makes little sense. A point to remember is your body has to service the muscle you build with nutrient rich blood. The development of unnecessary muscle will place additional load on the heart in a similar fashion to excess body fat. Be sensible in your approach and seek to develop your body to a pleasing and healthy level of functional muscularity. Unfortunately many body builders are not driven by a desire to achieve better health, but rather by a vain desire to impress others. To this end some individuals go to great lengths to achieve a level of gross muscularity, which puts at risk their health and future well-being.

MUSCLE BUILDING FOOD

Misinformation regarding our major source of energy has seen body builders stoking their bodies with massive amounts of carbohydrate. Fat is our major and most potent source of energy. As saturated fats have been embroiled in the controversy over cholesterol, increased carbohydrate consumption has been accompanied by a decrease in fat and protein intake. Apart from bone and a lot of water our bodies are constructed almost entirely of protein. Nothing else you eat will have any significant influence over the development of muscle.

You do not have to be overweight to benefit from the *Slim Forever* program. If you are happy with your present level of body fat you should go directly to the **weight maintenance** part of the program. This will preserve your level of body fat and enhance your energy producing and muscle building capabilities. Please refer to Chapter 1 *Your personal weight loss program* to establish your optimum daily requirements of both carbohydrate and protein.

Although your energy output will increase with exercise, the additional energy will come from stored and dietary fats. The heavier the exercise, the greater will be the shift in emphasis from carbohydrate to fat for energy. Under no circumstances should you increase your carbohydrate intake above the level indicated for your lean body weight. However, as you are seeking to build larger muscles the amount of protein you consume will have to increase. The greater the load you place on your body the greater will be your need for dietary protein and fat. As the amount of fat you consume is reasonably proportional to the amount of protein you eat, we only need to address the issue of protein.

The following calculations have been made on the assumption that the time you spend in the gymnasium is being used primarily in exercising. It is further assumed you are exercising within your safe limit, but you are increasing your exercise weights in accordance with your improving level of fitness.

Table 20.1 lists three exercise periods with varying durations in time. If you intend to gain muscle you will need to exercise for a minimum of 40 minutes each session with a minimum of three sessions each week. If you adopt a routine of less than these minimum requirements you will not succeed in increasing your muscle size. Be honest when assessing the time involved in your work-out periods. Protein consumed in excess of your actual requirements will only initiate the formation of unwanted body fat, not muscle.

The percentage increase in protein consumption is based on your optimum daily protein allowance according to your current lean body weight. For example, if your lean body weight is 168 lb/76 kg your optimum daily allowance of protein without exercise would be 17 oz/490 g. If your exercise sessions are of a duration of 50 minutes your daily protein allowance would increase by 45% to 25 oz/710 g. Or, if you exercise regularly for 60 to 80 minutes your daily protein allowance would increase by 50% to 26 oz/735 g, or 55% to 27 oz/760 g for exercise routines greater than 80 minutes duration. See Table 20.1.

The amount of additional protein you will require is not directly proportional to the time you spend exercising. Your ability to maintain constant exercise is greatest between 40 and 80 minutes. After 80 minutes your output curve will begin to fall and your rate of additional muscle gain will decline accordingly.

EXERCISE PERIOD (minutes)	PERCENTAGE INCREASE IN PROTEIN
40 – 60	Add 45%
60 – 80	Add 50%
Over 80	Add 55%

**Additional Protein Requirement
for Buiding Muscle
Table 20.1**

There is just one more rule that applies. You may only consume your appropriate level of increased protein for as many days as you exercise, plus one. That is to say, if you exercise three times a week you would consume additional protein four days each week. A four day routine would allow you to consume additional protein on five days each week, and so on. You should commence high protein intake on the day prior to your first exercise period for the week and then on the actual days you exercise. This will charge your body with protein in time to meet the demands of your first exercise routine and maintain it for the duration of your training week. For example, if you regularly exercise on Mondays, Wednesdays and Fridays you would consume your increased protein allowance on Sunday and again on each of your exercise days. On the days you do not exercise you must return to your base daily protein allowance to avoid consuming protein in excess of your requirements. The same rule applies to four and five day routines, but if you follow a six day routine you will of course be able to consume your increased protein requirement every day.

Protein intake during maintenance exercise

Your body requires more protein during muscle construction than it does during muscle maintenance. Once you reach your goal of muscle development you should reduce your daily intake of additional protein to the level stated in Table 20.2. Again these percentages are an expression of your lean body weight requirements.

EXERCISE PERIOD (minutes)	PERCENTAGE INCREASE IN PROTEIN
40 – 60	Add 20%
60 – 80	Add 27%
Over 80	Add 32%

**Additional Protein Requirement
for Muscle Maintenance
Table 20.2**

A word about using steroids and performance enhancing drugs

Don't.

The apparent short-term benefits of using anabolic steroids, hormones and other performance enhancing drugs are grossly outweighed by the long-term devastation they cause.

If we are to understand why these drugs are so dangerous we must first understand the effect they have on metabolic function. There are two distinct phases of metabolism. The first is the tissue building or anabolic phase, and the second is the tissue destruction or catabolic phase. Performance enhancers are usually anabolic in nature. That is to say they impose on the construction phase of overall metabolic function and body development. If you artificially increase anabolism over catabolism you must therefore increase overall body size, but cellular increase is not confined to the skeletal muscles.

Anabolic Steroids

Under the influence of anabolic stimulants almost every cell in the human body will become enlarged, and this can be extremely dangerous. Take, for example, the heart. Anabolic steroids do not cause a proportional enlargement of the heart, just a thickening of the muscular walls. As the heart walls thicken they protrude both outwardly and inwardly and reduce the capacity of the heart to hold blood. Decreased heart capacity will in turn lead to an increase in respiration rate and arterial hypertension. Increased body size and decreased blood pumping capacity combine to reduce overall physical performance due to a relative shortage of oxygenated blood. The onset of cardiac arrest, especially when a body is constantly exposed to heavy exercise, is a very real consideration with the taking of anabolic steroids.

Perhaps the organs most adversely affected by anabolic steroids are the kidneys and liver. These organs also increase in size but they become soft and mushy, unlike muscle which becomes harder and stronger. The necessity for dialysis treatment for failing kidneys, and the probability of kidney and liver transplants is becoming a stark reality in the world of drug taking body builders.

Growth hormone

Growth hormone has also become a fashionable body building drug. This very important hormone not only controls muscle and organ growth, it is also a major player in bone growth. Any pathological increase in the levels of growth hormone in the body gives rise to conditions known as giantism in the adolescent, and acromegaly in the adult. Giantism is typified by the excessive growth of the long bones of the body, such as those in the legs and arms, resulting in appendages which appear too long for the body. In the adult, the abnormal growth pattern is confined to the flat bones such as the skull, the jaw and the sternum. Body builders who take growth hormone become acromegalic and develop a noticeable enlargement of the forehead. The lower jaw becomes square and protrudes forward, and telltale gaps appear between the teeth. Although acromegalics are now living longer due to the administration of medication, former sufferers of this condition had a diminished projected life span of approximately 45 years.

Testosterone

The male hormone testosterone is used widely by both male and female body builders. Testosterone enhances body growth in both sexes but the side effects are dramatic. Following an initial period of increased sexual arousal, males suffer a loss of libido and potency with atrophy of the testes. Outwardly the female takes on distinct male characteristics such as the appearance of facial hair, a deeper voice and male muscularity. Less obvious is a decrease in sexual drive and an enlargement of the clitoris and labia majora, the female analogues of the male penis and testes. Just as the female hormone oestrogen will initiate breast development in the male, testosterone in the female will initiate the futile growth of male genitalia. Of concern to everyone around them, steroid taking body builders become extremely aggressive and exhibit mood swings involving periods of uncharacteristic bad temper.

While the taking of anabolic steroids will help build bigger and stronger muscles in the short-term, they cause demineralisation of bone which in turn can lead to the onset of a condition known as osteoporosis. The combination of a large strong body, weakened bones and heavy weights is a recipe for disaster.

The great irony of steroid and hormone abuse is that the effects do not last, just the destruction they cause. Enlarged muscles resulting from the taking of steroids cannot be sustained without ongoing substance abuse. In some reported cases massive muscle loss has been apparent even when anabolic steroids and hormones are being administered. Lives are being unnecessarily destroyed and lost by a practice that is both illegal and farcical.

Is there a better way?

Yes, there is a better way. Not only can you build a physique more pleasing to the eye, but you can do so while enhancing your health and well-being, not destroying it.

With the development of the *Slim Forever* program came an understanding of how and why muscles react positively to specific foods and exercise. By following the program presented in this text you can reach your desired goal of muscular fitness and live to enjoy it.

FAT OFF, MUSCLE ON

You may lose fat and gain muscle, but not effectively at the same time. If you are one of the many millions of people who are both overweight and under-muscled you can achieve your desired goal in one of three ways. By following the *Slim Forever* program you can:

1 reduce your unwanted body fat first and then concentrate on building muscle;

2 first concentrate on building muscle and then reduce your excess body fat; or

3 you can alternate between muscle gain and fat loss and achieve both goals simultaneously.

Options (1) and (2) are self-explanatory. However, if you adopt option (1) you may be disappointed to find how little muscle you have on your body once you lose those extra pounds. If you choose option (2) and seek to gain muscle in the presence of fat, the apparent fat content on your body will become exaggerated. On the other hand, option (3) has much to offer and is the recommended choice. By alternating between fat loss and muscle gain you can replace the amount of fat you lose with functional muscle and avoid appearing too thin, or even more overweight than you are at this moment.

If you choose option (3) you should coincide the weight loss and the muscle gain portions of your program with the phases of your physical biorhythm. Once you have established your physical biorhythmic cycle you may commence your program with a period of 34 days of muscle gain. This you will do by increasing your protein intake on the day your biorhythm crosses the line of neutrality as it travels from a negative cycle into a positive cycle. This is demonstrated in Figure 20.2.

By choosing this day as your starting point you will include two positive phases but only one negative phase. This will allow you to maximise your muscle gain potential in each alternate 34-day period.

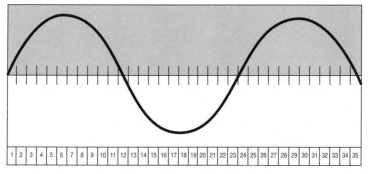

| 1 | 2 | 3 | 4 | 5 | 6 | 7 | 8 | 9 | 10 | 11 | 12 | 13 | 14 | 15 | 16 | 17 | 18 | 19 | 20 | 21 | 22 | 23 | 24 | 25 | 26 | 27 | 28 | 29 | 30 | 31 | 32 | 33 | 34 | 35 |

34-Day Muscle Gain Period
Figure 20.2

Once you complete your 34 days of muscle gain you will enter your first 35-day period of fat loss. This period will commence when your physical biorhythm crosses the line of neutrality from positive phase to negative phase as demonstrated in Figure 20.3.

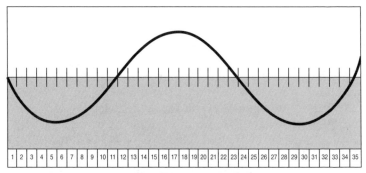

35-Day Fat Loss Period
Figure 20.3

Each of your 35-day periods of fat loss will occupy two negative cycles but only one positive cycle. This is to your advantage as your rate of fat loss will remain relatively constant during both the positive and negative cycles. Therefore, you will maximise your efforts by using two out of every three positive cycles for muscle gain, and two out of every three negative cycles for fat loss.

Repeat the process until you reach either your desired level of body fat or your desired level of muscularity. If these occur simultaneously you must immediately adopt the **weight maintenance** part of your program from Chapter 1, together with the appropriate increase in protein for muscle maintenance as outlined in this chapter.

If you reach your desired level of fat loss and still seek muscle gain, simply adopt your **weight maintenance** allowances and maintain full muscle building protein intake. Once you achieve total muscle growth you will continue with **weight maintenance** and reduce your protein intake to your appropriate muscle maintenance level.

If you reach full muscle growth before you achieve full fat reduction you must revert to your food allowances according to your **weight loss** assessment. If you persist with increased protein intake you will generate the production of glucose and you may negate the fat burning process. Once you reach both goals you may switch to **weight maintenance** and increase your muscle maintenance protein intake accordingly.

Should you at any time have the need to lose body fat or gain additional muscle or both, following either a lay-off from exercise or from **weight maintenance**, you would simply choose the appropriate course of action as outlined above.

At first glance this process may appear a little complicated, but in practice it is quite simple, but more importantly, *it works*. People who join health clubs and exercise to lose body fat or to gain muscle often become disillusioned and quit. You cannot lose unwanted body fat without initiating specific dietary change, nor can you gain muscle without exercising against resistance and increasing your intake of dietary protein.

Your pathway to success will be your *Slim Forever* program. If you take time now to embrace what it has to offer you will have the rest of your life to enjoy the results.

part III

THE WAY

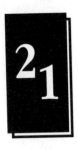

eat, drink and be slim

WHAT TO EAT

Y ou may eat anything you want provided you do not consume carbohydrate before your evening meal during **weight loss**, or exceed your daily carbohydrate and protein allowances.

The changes you will make in your eating habits will soon become part of your daily routine, changes which will be readily accepted by your body. You will find that within just a few weeks of starting this program many of the foods you could not previously do without will lose their appeal. A healthy body eating healthy food will soon treat food which is not nutritionally balanced as an unwelcome intruder.

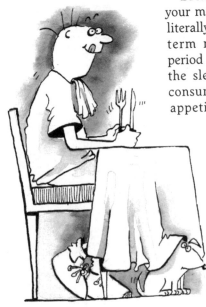

Breakfast and dinner will become your main meals of the day. Breakfast literally means 'breaking the fast', a term referring to the end of the period of going without food during the sleeping hours. As the protein consumed at breakfast satiates the appetite, lunch will be your least important meal, requiring only a protein snack to get you through to dinner or, you may choose the option of increasing the amount of protein you eat at breakfast and miss lunch altogether. The additional protein consumed in the morning will be sufficient to see you safely through to your evening meal without feeling hungry.

Breakfast

The choice of food available to you for breakfast is vast, and by combining ingredients you can develop an enormous collection of breakfast recipes. As you are limited to protein for breakfast during **weight loss**, eggs and meat will become your morning fare. However, as mushrooms are carbohydrate free and very versatile, you may eat as many as you want for breakfast. For example, consider eggs which you can have fried, boiled, poached, broasted, scrambled or made into an omelette. You can have them plain or with cheese, bacon, mushroom, ham, or with any number of these items in combination.

You may choose any form of meat, with the exception of liver which contains stored sugar in the form of glycogen. Your choices include steak, ground or minced beef patties, pork sausage, commercial sausage made without filler, pork or lamb chops, bacon or kidneys. You may eat the meat alone or in combination with an egg cooked to your liking, and perhaps mushrooms.

You may eat seafood for breakfast with such dishes as grilled fish with butter and just a squeeze of lemon, or perhaps steamed smoked cod with a poached egg. Prawns or leftover diced chicken scrambled with eggs with a few drops of soy sauce are also delicious.

Your choice of breakfast dishes will be limited only by your capacity for culinary adventure.

Lunch

If you eat breakfast, make lunch your snack meal. You may choose cold cuts of meat which could include ham, corned beef, salami, luncheon sausage made without filler, and leftover cold chicken. Cheese, especially tasty or matured cheese, is a great appetite suppressor and goes well with cold cuts.

You may choose seafood such as canned tuna or salmon which you may eat cold with mayonnaise, with a few drops of vinegar, or broiled with a little cheese topping. Grilled or steamed fish, fresh cooked prawns, Thai fish soup and poached smoked cod with butter are also tempting lunchtime snacks.

The lunch menu suggestions appearing in the next section contain recipes for American tuna, salmon and chicken salads which are all very tasty. They do contain a little onion, celery and parsley, which is of course carbohydrate, but they are added in such small amounts as to not be detrimental to your **weight loss** program.

Mushrooms are great for lunch and you may have them sautéed in butter, or stuffed and grilled with fillings such as ham, cheese or crabmeat. You may of course have any meat dish you desire for lunch, with the exception of liver during **weight loss**, or you have the option of choosing an item from the breakfast selection.

If you are planning on having a more formal luncheon, for example with friends or business associates, you may reduce your protein intake at breakfast and eat more during the day. There is no reason why you should feel deprived of good and satisfying food for your midday snack or meal.

Dinner

The sky is the limit at dinner, provided of course you do not exceed your daily intake allowances of either protein or carbohydrate. As you can now have carbohydrate, your choice of food becomes almost infinite.

You may eat any red meat, poultry, game, lamb, pork or veal dish you choose with any vegetable or combination of vegetables or salads. Because the *Slim Forever* program permits you to eat natural fats you can eat any salad dressing, provided it does not contain added sugar. You can make any number of delicious sauces, including those made with cream, and you may cook with wine if that is your fancy.

Due to the sheer magnitude of dinner selections, any attempt at listing the available options would fail in giving this subject the attention it deserves. You can eat simple meals such as steak with baked potato and salad, or you may choose to prepare more exotic meals such as those presented in the following section.

Living in the fast lane and throwing down food just to fill the void will soon take its toll. Slow down, eat well, and take full advantage of the enjoyment one of life's basic pleasures can bring.

WHAT TO DRINK

Many commercial diet programs concentrate on dictating what food a person should eat with little attention being given to choice of drinks. In many cases the drinks consumed may be a greater contributor to the formation of unwanted body fat than solid food.

As boring as it may seem, the human body requires the daily intake of just one liquid – water. The greater part of the human body is water, approximately 60% of total body weight in most cases. In real terms, if your total body weight is 150 lb/68 kg, the water content of your body will be in the vicinity of 90 lb/41 kg.

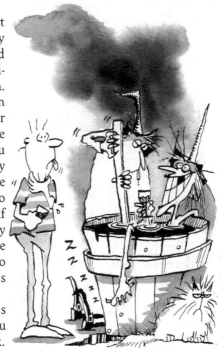

Your body will extract the water content of any drink you consume, and will deal with the additives the best way it can. However, even water can be heavily polluted, so for the sake of your health be selective in what you drink. A good test for any drink is to look at the glass before you put it to your lips and ask yourself – do I want this in my bloodstream? Because that is where it is going to be just a few minutes after you drink it.

Here are a few tips that may be of use to you in deciding what to drink.

Water

The only fluid the body requires, but beware of contaminated tap water. If there is any question as to the purity of the water you are drinking, either buy water from the supermarket, or purchase a water purifier.

Tea

Tea is made from the dried new leaves of the tea plant, but tea does contain both tannin and caffeine. However, there is good news for tea drinkers. Stassen Natural Foods Limited of Sri Lanka (Ceylon) produces and markets a tea which is organically grown without chemicals or pesticides, and is 98% caffeine free. The caffeine has been cultivated out of the tea and not removed after picking as is the case with decaffeinated coffee. The tea is mild to the taste but full of natural flavour and should satisfy even the most discerning of tea drinkers.

If tea is taken black, the tannin will be absorbed by the body, but the English tradition of adding milk overcomes rendering it harmless to the body. If you like your tea a little sweeter try either an artificial sweetener, during the day or perhaps a $\frac{1}{4}$ teaspoon of honey in the evening. Above all, avoid sugar.

Herbal teas are also available in a variety of flavours which do not require the addition of sweeteners. Herbal teas are relatively new to the market, and although some manufacturers claim their products to be health elixirs, the benefits, and for that matter the deficiencies, have yet to be established.

The following table lists the caffeine content of the various types of tea available.

TYPE OF TEA	CAFFEINE CONTENT (mg per 5 oz/150 ml cup)
Brewed	40 - 60
Instant	30
Caffeine reduced	0.6
Herbal	0

Caffeine Content of Tea
Table 21.1

Coffee

Much has been written to the detriment of coffee as a drink. Caffeine has been blamed for headaches, cardiac irregularities, breast cysts in females, cancer, peptic ulcers, diabetes, psychosis and even birth defects.

Of special interest to overweight people is that caffeine stimulates the pancreas to produce unwanted insulin. This surge of insulin accelerates the uptake of glucose from the bloodstream to the muscle cells, giving the coffee drinker a quick lift. However, it often reduces normal blood sugar levels to a point of hypoglycaemia. Coffee drinkers often experience the onset of headaches and light-headedness associated with low blood sugar which they usually overcome by eating something sweet, and on goes the body fat.

A point to remember is that 'good' can be enjoyable, but never addictive. An addiction occurs only when the normal chemistry of the body is altered. Caffeine is addictive and should be eliminated from the diet, or its intake severely restricted.

Decaffeinated coffee is available, but the chemicals used in the decaffeination process are extremely harmful. An alternate method of decaffeinating coffee employs the use of water, a process which is reported as being chemical free.

If you are on the **weight loss** part of your program you must avoid drinking coffee or drinks containing caffeine during the day. As caffeine stimulates the overproduction of insulin, the delicate balance of blood sugar necessary to lose body fat will be disrupted, and you will experience the onset of unnecessary hunger.

The following table lists the caffeine content of the various types of coffee available.

TYPE OF COFFEE	CAFFEINE CONTENT (mg per 5 oz/150 ml cup)
Brewed, drip method	115
percolated	80
Instant, non-decaffeinated	65
Decaffeinated, brewed	3
instant	2

Caffeine Content of Coffee
Table 21.2

Milk

Milk is an excellent food, but it does contain sugar in the form of lactose. A glass of milk contains approximately 8 g of carbohydrate, which is enough to negate the fat burning process if consumed during the day. You may drink milk in the evening provided you take the carbohydrate content into account when tallying your daily score.

Skimmed and fat reduced milks are marketed as the healthy alternatives, based on the assumption that fats are bad for us. Fat reduction results in the removal of healthy fats and the retention of the sugar content, so, if you choose to drink milk, drink it as Mother Nature intended it to be.

Soft drinks and pop

Here we have a real problem. The soft drink industry is booming, yet there is not one soft drink manufactured in the world that qualifies as being healthy. The basis of all soft drinks is sugar, water and carbon dioxide, to which is added flavouring, mostly artificial, and preservatives.

Diet drinks which are low in caffeine or are caffeine free and do not contain sugar may be consumed in moderation. But remember, soft drinks are totally devoid of nutrients and do contain chemical preservatives.

Fruit juices

Fruit juices are not the vitamin and mineral powerhouses they are thought to be. By comparison, fruit does not contain the concentrations of nutrients found in many vegetables, but does contain a lot more natural sugar. The early picking of a fruit while it is still green detracts greatly from its nutrient content. Many vitamins and minerals in fruit only reach full concentration with natural ripening, a maturation process which is not achieved when fruit is ripened artificially.

Vitamins and minerals are very susceptible to damage when exposed to light, and it is for this reason most vitamin and mineral manufacturers market their products in brown glass bottles or light-proof plastic containers. Fruit juice is usually marketed in clear glass or plastic containers to allow the purchaser to see the product, but this is done at the expense of much of what remains of the original nutrients.

Commercially produced fruit juice is often little more than sugar, water and natural flavourings. The process of juicing removes the cellulose content of the fruit which serves to concentrate the sugar. And, as a person may drink the juice of six oranges as opposed to eating just one orange, the increase in overall sugar consumption is greatly increased.

Fruit juice should be squeezed from fresh and naturally ripened fruit, and consumed immediately. As it contains a considerable amount of sugar, fruit juice should only be consumed in the evening during **weight loss**.

Beer

This ageless beverage does have a reputation for putting on weight. But, mouthful for mouthful, it contains less than one-third of the carbohydrate of most soft drinks and fruit juices. The drawback with beer is in the quantity consumed, as most beer drinkers down more than is necessary to quench the thirst.

A 12 oz/350 ml can of beer contains between 10 and 15 g of carbohydrate, depending on the brewer's recipe. However, the ardent beer drinker can still enjoy a can provided it is taken into consideration when assessing the daily carbohydrate intake.

Light beers tend to be a bit of a trap. The term light refers to the alcohol content and usually not to the sugar content of the beer. Light brews may be even higher in carbohydrate than their full alcohol cousins due to the additional use of sugar in the brewing process. Additional sugar is sometimes added to overcome the flat taste associated with some low alcohol beers.

Wine

The sugar content of table wine can vary considerably. Some varieties of grape yield a higher natural sugar content than others. Grapes picked late in the season are usually sweeter than the early harvest of the same grape, and grapes grown in drier regions tend to have a lower sugar content than grapes from wetter regions.

A glass of good quality dry wine will usually contain somewhere between 5 and 7 g of carbohydrate which can easily be assessed as part of your daily carbohydrate assessment allowance. You are encouraged with the *Slim Forever* program to enjoy, within reason, the foods and beverages that give you pleasure. If you subscribe to the adage that a meal without wine is like a day without sunshine, by all means go ahead and enjoy a glass, but only with your evening meal during **weight loss**. Many studies suggest it will do you more good than harm.

Spirits

Spirits tend to be low in carbohydrate and can be enjoyed in moderation in the evening during weight loss, provided what you mix with the spirit is not high in carbohydrate. Mixes with water, mineral water, soda water and limited amounts of fruit juice and diet soft drinks are acceptable. But, high carbohydrate mixes such as tonic water, bitter lemon, Coca-Cola, dry ginger ale and Tom Collins mix should be taken in absolute moderation.

In summary

Drinks containing carbohydrate or caffeine should not be consumed until just prior to, during, or immediately after your evening meal, and then only in moderation.

During the day you may have unlimited quantities of fresh water, mineral water or soda water. Water-decaffeinated coffee and 98% caffeine free tea taken with milk, with or without artificial sweetener, and herbal teas are acceptable day and night drinks.

Low carbohydrate content alcohol drinks may be consumed but not until the sun is well over the yardarm, which in this case is just prior to, during, or immediately following the evening meal. There is, however, a warning that comes with consuming alcohol during **weight loss**. As your body will continue in its hypoglycaemic state until after the carbohydrate from the evening meal reaches the bloodstream, greater than two drinks may initiate the onset of a hangover. Even mild and controlled hypoglycaemia renders the body more susceptible to the effects of alcohol, so practise moderation and savour the enjoyment without the discomfort.

cooking the slim forever way

The *Slim Forever* program is *not* a diet. It does not require you to eat any special food, other than to reduce your carbohydrate intake and balance what you are already eating.

This is not a cook book. It is a collection of recipes which will assist you in understanding just how adventurous you can be with your selection of food. The following pages contain menu suggestions for breakfast, lunch and dinner, including salad dressings, soups and appetisers.

Each recipe has been adapted to produce servings of average size. The number of servings, together with the protein and carbohydrate content of each serving is indicated at the beginning of each recipe. You may wish to alter the size of the servings to suit your own requirements. This you can do by simply serving more or less of the suggested portions, or by increasing or decreasing the volume of all of the ingredients.

These recipes have been selected according to balance of nutrients, taste and ease of preparation. Be adventurous in your selection of meals and develop your own collection of balanced recipes. Eating with the *Slim Forever* program can, and should, be satisfying and fun.

Some of the breakfast and lunch recipes contain onion, parsley and chilli, but they are in such small amounts as to not register any adverse effect on weight loss. Treat any carbohydrate assessment bearing the word *trace* as being no carbohydrate.

The following abbreviations appear in the recipes in this section.

$$\begin{aligned}
\text{TBL} &\rightarrow \text{tablespoon} \\
\text{tsp} &\rightarrow \text{teaspoon} \\
\text{cup} &\rightarrow \text{8 fl oz/240 ml}
\end{aligned}$$

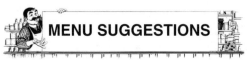

MENU SUGGESTIONS

APPETISERS

SEAFOOD

CHICKEN

PORK AND VEAL

LAMB

BEEF

Healthy eating the *Slim Forever* way ▶

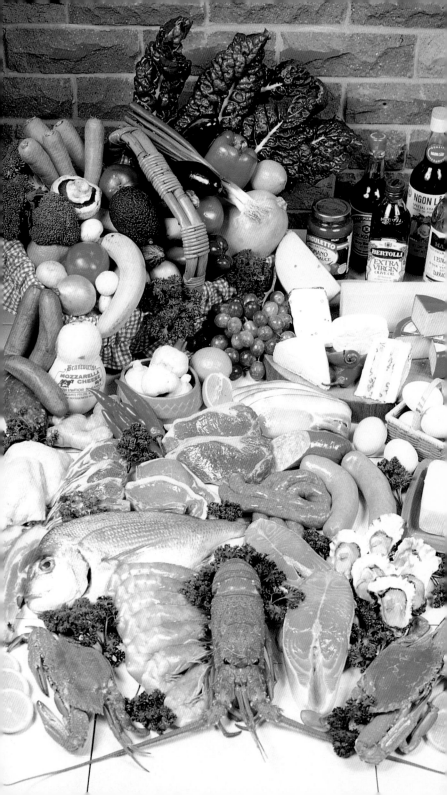

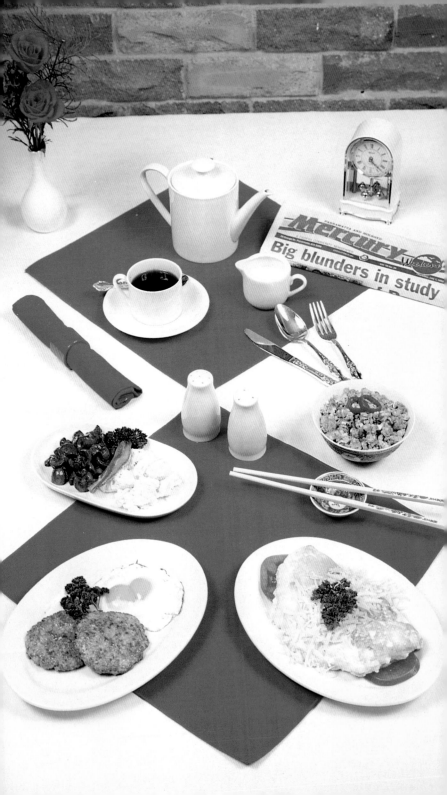

BREAKFAST

COUNTRY PORK SAUSAGE

Servings
4

Protein per serving..........4 oz/110 g
Carbohydrate per serving..........trace

**1 lb/450 g ground/minced
lean pork**

¾ tsp black pepper

⅓ tsp nutmeg, ground

¼ tsp sage, powdered

¼ tsp curry powder

Salt to taste

➪Combine all ingredients in
a mixing bowl and form into
8 patties.

➪Fry sausage patties in a
skillet or pan moistened
with butter until golden
brown on both sides. Serve.

Note: Patties may be frozen
for later use.

SCRAMBLED EGGS

Servings
1

Protein per serving.............3 oz/90 g
Carbohydrate per serving..........trace

2 eggs, large

2 TBL milk

1 tsp butter

Salt and pepper to taste

For suggested fillings please
refer to 'basic omelette'.
Filling not included in
nutrient assessment.

➪Beat eggs, milk, salt and
pepper in mixing bowl.

➪Melt butter in small
saucepan and add filling if
applicable.

➪Cover and cook over low
heat until egg mixture sets.

◀◀ Breakfast Dishes clockwise from left front.
1. Country pork sausage with egg 2. Devilled kidneys with
scrambled egg. 3. Pork stir-fry 4. Omelette with cheese.

PORK STIRFRY

Servings
1

Protein per serving.......4.5 oz/125 g
Carbohydrate per serving...........trace

3 oz/85 g ground/minced
    lean pork

1 tsp sesame oil

½ clove garlic, crushed

½ red chilli, seeded and chopped
    (optional)

Black pepper to taste

½ tsp soy sauce

½ tsp oyster sauce

½ tsp fish sauce (nam pla)

1 egg, beaten

⇨Heat oil in skillet or pan. Add garlic, chilli and pork and cook until pork is pale pink. Do not overcook or pork will dry out.

⇨Add pepper, soy, oyster and fish sauces and cook for 1 minute.

⇨Add beaten egg, stir, and cook until egg sets. Serve immediately.

CHEESY EGGS

Servings
1

Protein per serving..........4 oz/110 g
Carbohydrate per serving...........trace

2 eggs, large

½ tsp butter

1 oz/30 g tasty cheese, shredded

⇨Heat butter in skillet or pan. Add eggs and cook until white begins to set.

⇨Sprinkle cheese over eggs, cook for 1 minute, turn and continue cooking until cheese is golden brown. Or,

⇨Cover eggs with lid and cook until eggs are set and cheese is melted. Serve.

DEVILLED KIDNEYS

Servings
1

Protein per serving.......3.5 oz/100 g
Carbohydrate per serving...........trace

**2 lamb kidneys or 3.5 oz/100 g
calves kidney**

1 tsp butter

¼ tsp garlic, crushed

➪Remove membrane and fat from kidneys and cut into bite sized pieces.

➪Soak kidneys in cold salty water for 30 minutes. Drain.

➪Melt butter in skillet or pan, add garlic and kidneys and sauté until just cooked through.

➪Serve kidneys topped with juices from pan.

OMELETTE

Servings
1

Protein per serving.............3 oz/90 g
Carbohydrate per serving...........trace

2 eggs, large

1 tsp butter

Salt and pepper to taste

Suggested fillings*

Shredded cheese
Sautéed mushrooms
Grilled bacon pieces
Diced ham
Diced chicken
Cooked prawns
Crabmeat

(*not included in nutrient assessment)

➪Separate eggs and beat whites until stiff. Lightly beat yolks and stir gently into whites with salt and pepper.

➪Melt butter in skillet or pan over medium heat. Add egg mixture and cook until golden brown on bottom.

➪Place pan under broiler or griller until omelette sets and is golden brown. Serve flat or folded in half. Or, place filling on one-half of omelette, fold in half and cook over low heat until egg sets, turning once. Serve.

LUNCH

BEEF PATTY MELT

Servings
1

Protein per serving..........4 oz/110 g
Carbohydrate per serving...........trace

3 oz/90 g ground/minced lean beef	▷Combine meat, onion, parsley, salt and pepper and form into patty.
½ tsp onion, chopped	
¼ tsp parsley, chopped	▷Melt butter in skillet or pan and fry patty on both sides until brown.
Salt and pepper to taste	
½ tsp butter	▷Remove patty from pan and place in an ovenproof dish. Top with cheese and broil grill until cheese melts. Serve.
1 oz/30 g tasty cheese	

LEMON CHICKEN KEBABS

Servings
2

Protein per serving..........4 oz/110 g
Carbohydrate per serving...........trace

8 oz/225 g boneless chicken breast cut into cubes	▷Combine all ingredients in a bowl and refrigerate for 2 hours.
1 tsp olive oil	
½ TBL lemon juice	▷Thread chicken pieces onto a skewer and broil or grill until chicken is cooked and lightly browned. Serve.
2 drops Tobasco sauce	
Pinch dried taragon	
Salt and pepper to taste	

THAI FISH CAKES

Servings
5

Protein per serving..........4 oz/110 g
Carbohydrate per serving..........trace

1 lb/450 g white fish with skin and bone removed

½ tsp fresh coriander leaves, chopped

¼ tsp curry powder

1 egg

1 garlic clove, crushed

1 red chilli, seeded and chopped

Black pepper to taste

1½ TBL fish sauce (nam pla)

2 TBL sesame or olive oil

▷Combine all ingredients except oil in mixing bowl and refrigerate for 90 minutes.

▷Heat oil in skillet or pan and spoon fish mixture directly into pan forming small flat patties.

▷Cook for 2 minutes or until fish is lightly browned on both sides. Serve.

MUSHROOMS STUFFED WITH HAM AND CHEESE

Servings
1

Protein per serving............3 oz/90 g
Carbohydrate per serving..........trace

2 or 3 large mushrooms

1 tsp butter

½ tsp onion, chopped

⅛ tsp garlic, crushed

2 oz/60 g ham, diced

Salt and pepper to taste

1 oz/30 g tasty cheese, shredded

▷Remove stems from mushrooms. Heat butter in skillet or pan and sauté mushroom caps for 1½ minutes each side. Remove from pan.

▷Chop mushroom stems and saute with onion, garlic, ham, salt and pepper for 2 minutes.

▷ Place mushroom caps, skin side down, in an ovenproof dish and stuff with mixture. Top with cheese and broil or grill till cheese melts.

AMERICAN CHICKEN, TUNA OR SALMON SALAD

Servings	Protein per serving.......3.5 oz/100 g
2	Carbohydrate per serving...........trace

6 oz /170 g of cooked chopped chicken, tuna or salmon.	⇨Combine all ingredients in a mixing bowl.
1 tsp celery, finely chopped	⇨Refrigerate and serve.
1 tsp onion, finely chopped	
½ tsp parsley, chopped	
1 egg, hard boiled, chopped	
1½ TBL mayonnaise	
½ TBL sour cream	
Salt and pepper to taste	

QUICK TUNA AND CHEESE CASSEROLE

Servings	Protein per serving..........4 oz/110 g
1	Carbohydrate per serving...........trace

3 oz/60 g tuna, drained	⇨Combine tuna, onion, parsley, salt and pepper and place in small ovenproof dish.
1 tsp onion, finely chopped	
½ tsp parsley, chopped	⇨Top with cheese and bake in oven for 10 minutes.
Salt and pepper to taste	
1 oz/30 g tasty cheese, shredded	⇨Grill or broil until cheese forms golden bubbles and serve.

Lunch dishes clockwise from centre front.   ▶▶
1. Beef patty melt 2. Lemon chicken kebabs
3. Thai fish cakes 4. Mushrooms stuffed with ham and cheese
5. Cheese and meat platter 6. American chicken salad.

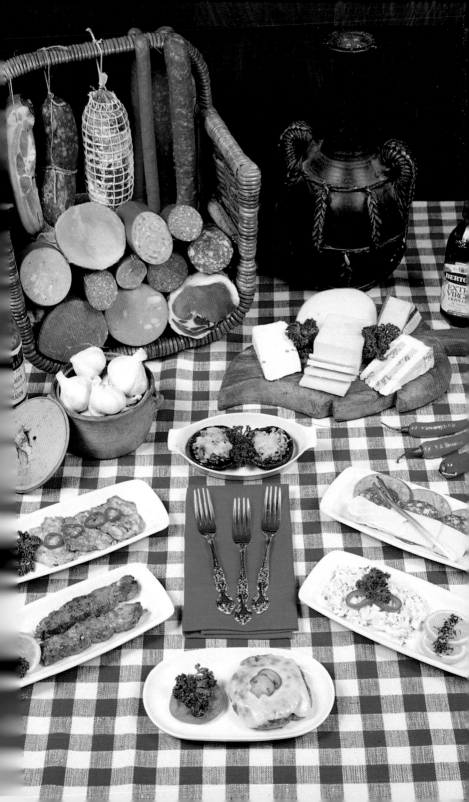

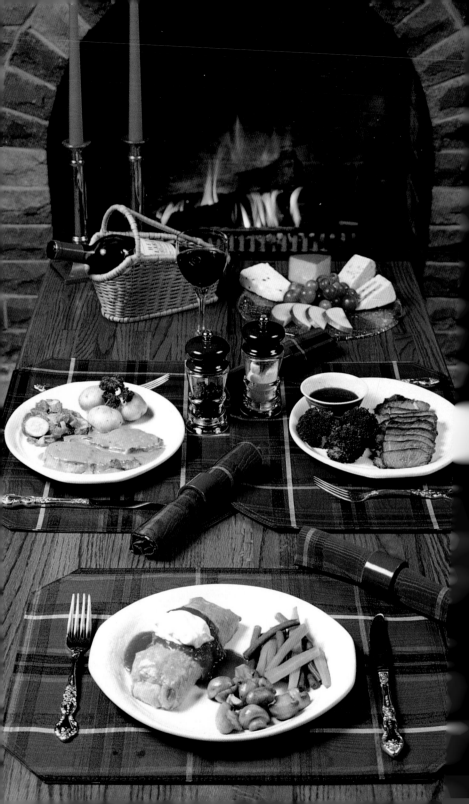

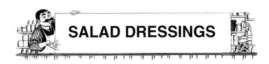

SALAD DRESSINGS

CREAMY RANCH DRESSING

Servings
4

Protein per serving.........0.5 oz/15 g
Carbohydrate per serving.................0

½ cup mayonnaise

½ cup sour cream

¼ tsp garlic

¼ tsp dried basil leaves

¼ tsp dried oregano

Parsley sprig

Salt and pepper to taste

⇨Combine all ingredients in blender and blend to a smooth consistency.

⇨Chill and serve.

GREEN GODDESS DRESSING

Servings
4

Protein per serving.........0.5 oz/15 g
Carbohydrate per serving.............1 g

¾ cup mayonnaise

¼ cup sour cream

1 green onion/shallot

½ garlic clove

½ TBL lemon juice

½ TBL tarragon vinegar

4 parsley sprigs

⇨Combine all ingredients in blender and blend to a smooth consistency.

⇨Chill and serve.

◀◀ Dinner dishes clockwise from front.
1. Italian chicken in fillo pastry 2. Bavarian pork chops
3. Oriental sliced beef.

CAESAR DRESSING

Servings
4

Protein per serving.........0.5 oz/15 g
Carbohydrate per serving..............1 g

½ cup olive oil

1 garlic clove

1 egg, lightly boiled

2 TBL lemon juice

1 tsp Worcestershire sauce

1 TBL tarragon vinegar

2 anchovy fillets

¼ cup parmesan cheese, grated

Fresh black pepper to taste

⇨ Combine all ingredients in blender.

⇨ Chill and serve.

ITALIAN DRESSING

Servings
4

Protein per serving............................0
Carbohydrate per serving..............1 g

¼ cup wine vinegar

1 tsp mustard powder

1 cup olive oil

2 garlic cloves

1 tsp dried oregano

½ tsp honey

Parsley sprig

Salt and pepper to taste

⇨ Combine ingredients in blender.

⇨ Chill and serve.

THOUSAND ISLAND DRESSING

Servings
4

Protein per serving............................0
Carbohydrate per serving.............2 g

¾ cup mayonnaise

¼ cup sweet chilli sauce

1 green onion/shallot

½ tsp capers

2 gherkins

2 parsley sprigs

½ TBL green bell pepper/capsicum

¼ tsp paprika

1 egg, hard boiled

↪ Combine mayonnaise, chilli sauce and paprika in mixing bowl.

↪ Finely chop all remaining ingredients.

↪ Blend with mayonnaise.

↪ Chill and serve.

BLUE CHEESE DRESSING

Servings
4

Protein per serving.........0.5 oz/15 g
Carbohydrate per serving..........trace

2 oz/60 g blue cheese

¼ cup sour cream

¼ cup mayonnaise

¼ cup cultured butter milk

Parsley sprig

Black pepper to taste

↪ Combine all ingredients in blender and blend to a smooth consistency.

↪ Chill to thicken before serving.

SOUPS

CHICKEN AND ASPARAGUS EGG DROP SOUP

Servings
4

Protein per serving.........1.5 oz/45 g
Carbohydrate per serving..............3 g

4 oz/110 g cooked chicken, diced

4 cups chicken stock

4 oz/110 g green asparagus tips, canned

2 eggs, lightly beaten

2 green onions/shallots, chopped

1 TBL corn starch mixed with water

⅛ tsp ground black pepper

Salt to taste

⮂ Place chicken stock, chopped chicken and asparagus in saucepan and bring to boil.

⮂ Reduce heat. Stir and slowly add corn starch.

⮂ Continue stirring and slowly add beaten eggs.

⮂ Season with salt and pepper, serve and garnish with chopped green onions.

FRENCH CREAM OF MUSHROOM SOUP

Servings
4

Protein per serving............................0
Carbohydrate per serving.............3 g

12 oz/350 g fresh mushrooms, sliced

2 oz/60 g butter

3 TBL plain flour

4 cups chicken stock

1 TBL lemon juice

⅔ cup thick cream

Salt and pepper to taste

⮂ Melt butter in saucepan and add flour stirring for 3 to 4 minutes. Do not brown.

⮂ Remove from heat, stir and slowly add chicken stock.

⮂ Return to heat bring to boil while continuing to stir.

⮂ Reduce heat and add lemon juice, mushrooms. Simmer 5 minutes.

⮂ Cool and purée in blender.

Parsley, chopped	⇨ Return to low heat and add cream, salt, pepper and nutmeg.
Pinch nutmeg	
	⇨ Serve and garnish with chopped parsley.

THAI SEAFOOD SOUP

Servings	Protein per serving..........4 oz/110 g
4	Carbohydrate per serving...........trace

1 lb/450 g uncooked mixed seafood (fish, squid, scallops, prawns)	⇨Place chicken stock, fish sauce, soy sauce, garlic, coriander and chilli in saucepan and bring to boil.
4 cups chicken stock	
1 TBL fish sauce (nam pla)	⇨Add seafood, cover and bring to boil. Simmer for 2 minutes.
1 tsp light soy sauce	
2 garlic cloves, minced	⇨Add salt and pepper and serve immediately.
1 tsp coriander leaves, chopped	
1 fresh red chilli, seeded & chopped	
Salt and pepper to taste	

MEXICAN CHICKEN SOUP

Servings	Protein per serving............1 oz/30 g
4	Carbohydrate per serving.............3 g

1 TBL olive oil	⇨Heat olive oil in saucepan and sauté onion until tender. Do not brown.
½ cup spanish onion, sliced	
4 cups chicken stock	⇨Add stock, salt and pepper and simmer chicken breast for 15 minutes or until tender.
4 oz/100 g chicken breast	

Salt and pepper to taste

4 TBL tomato puree/paste

½ cup thick cream

½ avocado pear, diced

Parsley or chives, chopped

⇨Remove chicken and cut into small cubes.

⇨Strain stock and save. Discard residue.

⇨Reheat stock, add tomato puree and simmer 15 minutes.

⇨Remove from heat and add chicken, cream and avocado.

⇨Serve and garnish with parsley or chives.

CREAM OF PUMPKIN SOUP

Servings 4

Protein per serving............................0
Carbohydrate per serving..........5.5 g

1½ oz/40 g butter

1 small onion, chopped

1 lb/450 g pumpkin, cooked and mashed

4 cups chicken stock

1½ cups milk

⅛ tsp all spice

⅛ tsp tabasco or chilli sauce

½ cup thick cream

Salt and pepper to taste

⇨Melt butter in saucepan and sauté onion until soft. Do not brown.

⇨Add all ingredients except cream and simmer for 15 minutes.

⇨Cool and puree in blender.

⇨Reheat but do not boil. Add cream.

⇨Serve hot or chilled.

LUMBERJACK CHEESE SOUP

Servings
4

Protein per serving.........1.5 oz/45 g
Carbohydrate per serving..........5.5 g

1½ oz/40 g butter

¼ cup carrot, finely chopped

¼ cup celery, finely chopped

¼ cup onion, finely chopped

1 TBL all purpose/plain flour

1½ cups milk

1½ cups chicken stock

Pinch paprika

1 cup sharp cheddar cheese,
shredded

Green onion, finely chopped

⇨Melt butter in saucepan. Add carrot, celery and onion and cook until tender. Do not brown.

⇨Add flour and stir for 2 minutes. Do not brown.

⇨Stir continually and add milk and chicken stock.

⇨Season with salt, pepper and paprika.

⇨Increase heat and stir until thick and bubbling.

⇨Reduce heat and stir in cheese until it melts. Do not boil.

⇨Serve and garnish with green onion.

APPETISERS

AVOCADO CRAB LOUIS

Servings   Protein per serving.............1 oz/30 g
  2   Carbohydrate per serving..............4 g

---

1 ripe avocado, halved and seeded

⮞Combine Sauce Louis ingredients in small bowl.

2 oz/60 g crabmeat, cooked

⮞Add crabmeat.

Sauce Louis

⮞Spoon into avocado halves.

2 TBL mayonnaise

⮞Chill and serve.

1 TBL sour cream

1 tsp sweet chilli sauce

⅛ tsp Worcestershire sauce

1 tsp green bell pepper/capsicum, finely chopped

1 tsp green onion/shallot, chopped

½ tsp lemon juice

Salt and pepper to taste

RUSSIAN EGGS

Servings   Protein per serving.............2 oz/60 g
  2   Carbohydrate per serving..........trace

---

2 eggs, hard boiled and chilled

⮞Cut eggs in half along their length and arrange cut side down on two serving dishes.

2 TBL mayonnaise

1 TBL sour cream

⮞Mix mayonnaise and sour cream together and spoon over eggs.

2 tsp caviar

2 lemon wedges	⇨Top with caviar.
2 parsley sprigs	⇨Garnish with lemon wedge and parsley.

ITALIAN CRABMEAT PATTIES

Servings 4	Protein per serving.............3 oz/90 g Carbohydrate per serving..........0.5 g
8 oz/220 g crab meat, cooked	⇨Combine crabmeat, garlic, parmesan cheese, egg, salt and pepper in a mixing bowl.
1 garlic clove, minced	
½ cup parmesan cheese, grated	⇨Form into small patties.
½ TBL parsley, chopped	⇨Heat oil in skillet or pan and cook patties on each side until golden brown.
1 egg	
Salt and pepper to taste	⇨Garnish with lemon wedge and parsley.
¼ cup olive oil	
4 lemon wedges	
4 parsley sprigs	

SESAME CHICKEN PIECES WITH GINGER

Servings 4	Protein per serving.............2 oz/60 g Carbohydrate per serving..........3.5 g
8 oz/220 g chicken breast, boned and cut into bite size pieces	⇨Combine chicken pieces, garlic, ginger, soy sauce, honey and sherry in a mixing bowl.
1 garlic clove, crushed	
2 TBL soy sauce	⇨Cover and refrigerate for 2 hours.
1 TBL ginger root, crushed	⇨Heat sesame oil in skillet or pan.
½ TBL honey	

1 TBL dry sherry	⇨Drain chicken and discard marinade.
2 TBL sesame oil	⇨Sauté chicken pieces over medium heat until tender.
1 tsp sesame seeds	⇨Sprinkle with sesame seeds and cook 2 minutes.
	⇨Serve as individual appetisers of as hors d'oeuvres speared with toothpicks.

SPANISH GARLIC PRAWNS

Servings	Protein per serving.............3 oz/90 g
2	Carbohydrate per serving..........0.5 g

8 king prawns, large, raw	⇨Remove head and shell from prawn leaving the tip of tail intact.
$\frac{1}{4}$ cup olive oil	⇨With a sharp knife cut prawn tail along its length to a depth of half its thickness. Devein and rinse.
2 oz/60 g butter	
4 garlic cloves, crushed	
1 red chilli, seeded and chopped (optional)	⇨Heat oil and butter in a saucepan. Add garlic, chilli, tomato, bell pepper and green onion. Simmer for 2 minutes.
1 TBL tomato, fresh, diced	
1 TBL red bell pepper/capsicum, diced	
1 TBL green onion/shallot, chopped	⇨Add prawns and raise heat to high. Cover and cook until prawns go opaque, about 3 minutes.
	⇨Arrange prawns in small deep bowls and cover with garlic butter sauce.

CHICKEN LIVER PÂTÉ

Servings	Protein per serving.........2.5 oz/70 g
4	Carbohydrate per serving..........0.5 g

2 oz/60 g butter	⇨Melt butter in saucepan. Add onion and bacon and sauté 3 minutes.
1 TBL onion, chopped	
2 oz/60 g bacon, chopped	⇨Add mushrooms and sauté 1 minute.
2 oz/60 g mushrooms, chopped	
¼ tsp thyme	⇨Add thyme, bayleaf and chicken livers. Stir and saute until livers are cooked but still pink.
1 bay leaf	
8 oz/225 g chicken livers	⇨Remove from heat and discard bay leaf. Combine livers, cream and brandy and blend until smooth.
¼ cup cream	
1 TBL brandy	⇨Spoon into mould and chill until set.
Salt and pepper to taste	

SEAFOOD

PAN FRIED FILLETS OF FISH

Servings
2

Protein per serving..........8 oz/225 g
Carbohydrate per serving..............5 g

1 lb/450 g fish fillets

½ cup all purpose/plain flour

¼ cup milk

1 egg

½ cup olive oil

⇨ Lightly beat egg and milk together in a bowl.

⇨ Heat oil in skillet or pan on low heat.

⇨ Dredge fish in flour and wash in egg mixture.

⇨ Again dredge fish in flour fry on both sides at low heat until golden brown.

Mayonnaise and Lemon Sauce

¼ cup mayonnaise

1 TBL lemon juice

1 tsp parsley, chopped

⇨ Combine ingredients in a small bowl and spoon over cooked fish fillets.

Spicy Mexican Sauce

2 oz/60 g butter

1 TBL red bell pepper/capsicum, finely diced

1 TBL green onion, chopped

2 garlic cloves, crushed

1 red chilli, seeded and chopped

1 tsp parsley, chopped

⇨ Melt butter in small saucepan over medium heat.

⇨ Add remaining ingredients and simmer for 4 minutes.

⇨ Spoon over cooked fish fillets.

SEAFOOD CIOPPINO

Servings
2

Protein per serving..........8 oz/225 g
Carbohydrate per serving..............8 g

1 TBL olive oil	⊳Heat oil in large saucepan. Sauté onions and garlic until tender. Do not brown.
½ medium onion, chopped	
1 garlic clove, crushed	⊳Add spices and simmer for 5 minutes.
Pinch oregano	
Pinch sage	⊳Add tomatoes, tomato paste, water, salt and pepper and simmer covered for 1 hour.
1 bay leaf	
12 oz/375 g tomatoes, canned, peeled	⊳Strain sauce and discard residue.
¼ TBL tomato paste	⊳Reheat sauce and add seafood. Cover and simmer 5 minutes.
⅛ cup water	
Salt and pepper to taste	⊳Serve in individual bowls.
1 lb/450 g mixed seafood (fish, prawns, mussels, calamari, crab etc)	

SALMON CROQUETTES

Servings
2

Protein per serving..........8 oz/225 g
Carbohydrate per serving..............6 g

14 oz/400 g pink salmon, canned	⊳Drain juice from salmon and reserve.
1 small onion, finely chopped	⊳Combine salmon, onion, parsley, potato, egg, salt and pepper in mixing bowl.
1 tsp parsley, finely chopped	
½ cup potato, boiled, mashed	⊳Heat oil in skillet or pan.
1 egg	

Salt and pepper to taste

¼ cup all purpose/plain flour

¼ cup olive oil

Butter Sauce

Salmon juice

¼ cup water

2 TBL white vinegar

1 tsp dill seed

1 red chilli, seeded and chopped
(optional)

2 oz/60 g butter

½ TBL corn starch/flour
mixed in cold water

⇨Form salmon mixture into
patties, roll in flour and
fry gently on both sides
until golden brown.

⇨Combine all ingredients
except flour in a small
saucepan.

⇨Bring to boil and simmer
for 3 minutes.

⇨Stir and thicken with corn
starch/flour.

⇨Spoon over salmon
croquettes.

CREAMED CURRIED PRAWNS

Servings
2

Protein per serving.........8 oz/ 225 g
Carbohydrate per serving.............6 g

1 lb/440 g prawns, large raw

1 TBL olive oil

1 oz/30 g butter

½ onion, medium, sliced

1 garlic clove, crushed

2 tsp curry powder (or to taste)

⇨Shell and devein prawns.

⇨Heat butter and olive oil
in medium saucepan. Add
onion and garlic and sauté
3 minutes. Do not brown.

⇨Add curry powder and chilli
and stir over very low heat
for 3 minutes.

⇨Add chicken stock. Increase
heat, cover, and simmer for
5 minutes.

½ red bell pepper/capsicum sliced

¾ cup chicken stock

1 red chilli, seeded, chopped

1 tsp parsley, chopped

Salt and pepper to taste

½ cup thick cream

½ TBL corn starch/flour mixed
    with cold water

⇨Add bell pepper/capsicum,
parsley and cream and bring
to boil.

⇨Add prawns and cook for 3
minutes or until prawns are
opaque.

⇨Thicken with corn starch/
flour and serve with
rice (not included in
carbohydrate assessment).

CHICKEN

FRENCH CHICKEN CASSEROLE

Servings
3

Protein per serving..........8 oz/225 g
Carbohydrate per serving...............5 g

2 lb/1 kg chicken, halved

1 garlic clove, crushed

¼ tsp tarragon, dried

⅛ tsp sage, dried

6 small onions, peeled

4 oz/120 g mushrooms, sliced

¾ cup celery, sliced

1 oz/30 g butter, melted

Wine Sauce

2 oz/60 g butter

1½ TBL all purpose/plain flour

Salt and pepper to taste

¾ cup chicken stock

¼ cup milk

⅛ cup dry white wine

¼ cup cream

⇨Place chicken halves in foil-lined baking dish. Sprinkle with garlic and herbs and bake in moderate oven for 20 minutes.

⇨Baste with melted butter and bake a further 20 minutes.

⇨Simmer onions in water for 5 minutes, remove and sauté in 1 oz/30 g butter until golden brown.

⇨Remove onion and sauté mushrooms until tender. Remove from pan.

⇨Add remaining butter to pan and add flour, salt and pepper. Stir for 3 minutes.

⇨Remove from heat, stir and gently add chicken stock, milk, cream and wine. Return to heat and simmer for 5 minutes.

⇨Joint cooked chicken and arrange in casserole dish. Add mushrooms, celery, onions, and sauce. Cover and bake in moderate oven for 20 minutes.

ITALIAN CHICKEN IN FILO PASTRY

Servings	Protein per serving.......7.5 oz/210 g
2	Carbohydrate per serving...........15 g

12 oz/340 g chicken breast, chopped

¼ tsp oregano, dried

¼ tsp basil, dried

2 oz/60 g camembert cheese, sliced

1 egg

1 tsp parsley, chopped

Salt and pepper to taste

3 sheets filo pastry

2 TBL prepared Italian tomato sauce

1 TBL sour cream

Accompany With

Steamed beans and sautéd mushrooms (not included in nutrient assessment)

➪Combine chicken, herbs, salt, pepper and parsley in mixing bowl.

➪Separate egg and reserve white. Add yolk to chicken mixture and stir.

➪Lay one sheet of pastry on bench and brush with melted butter. Lay second sheet on top and brush with butter.

➪Lay third sheet on top and cut pastry into two equal squares approximately 10 in x 10 in/25 cm x 25 cm.

➪Halve chicken mixture and lay it diagonally across pastry squares. Add camembert cheese, roll into envelopes and seal with beaten egg white.

➪Brush top of envelope with beaten egg white and bake on greased tray in moderate oven for 35 minutes or until golden brown.

➪Serve topped with warm tomato sauce and sour cream.

CURRIED CHICKEN WITH YOGHURT

Servings   Protein per serving..........8 oz/225 g
   3   Carbohydrate per serving.............6 g

2 lb/1 kg chicken, jointed

⅓ tsp black pepper, turmeric, cumin,
      chilli powder, cardamom
      cloves, cinnamon and mace

2 garlic cloves, crushed

1 tsp salt

2 TBL yoghurt

3 TBL olive oil

1 medium onion, sliced

1 cup chicken stock or water

▷ Combine all ingredients
except oil, onion and stock
in mixing bowl coating
chicken well with mixture.

▷ Heat oil in large saucepan
and gently fry onions until
tender. Do not brown.

▷ Add chicken and stir for 4
minutes. Add chicken stock
or water and cover.
Simmer for 90 minutes or
until chicken is tender.

▷ Serve with boiled rice (not
included in nutritional
assessment).

MALAYSIAN STEAMED CHICKEN

Servings   Protein per serving..........8 oz/225 g
   3   Carbohydrate per serving.............8 g

2 lb/1 kg chicken, jointed

3 TBL soy sauce

1 TBL oyster sauce

1 TBL fish sauce (nam pla)

1 TBL honey, melted

2 garlic cloves, crushed

½ tsp ginger root, chopped

½ cup olive oil

8 oz/220 g steamed broccoli

▷ Combine all ingredients
except oil in a bowl and
marinate for 2 hours.

▷ Heat oil in skillet or pan
and lightly fry chicken
pieces but do not cook.

▷ Place chicken in covered
saucepan and simmer 25
minutes or until cooked.

▷ Serve with steamed broccoli
using skimmed sauce as a
dip.

PORK AND VEAL

MEDALLIONS OF PORK ROSEMARY

Servings
2

Protein per serving..........8 oz/225 g
Carbohydrate per serving.............4 g

1 lb/450 g lean pork loin or fillet

2 TBL olive oil

1 garlic clove, crushed

½ cup dry white wine

¼ teaspoon rosemary, dried

Salt and pepper to taste

½ cup cream

⇨Cut pork into medallions and remove all fat.

⇨Heat oil in skillet or pan and sauté pork until cooked and slightly brown. Remove pork from pan and keep hot in oven.

⇨Lightly fry garlic in pan and add wine, rosemary, salt and pepper. Reduce wine by half and add cream.

⇨Return pork to pan including any juice that may have accumulated. Simmer for 3 minutes and serve.

PORK CHOPS WITH ORANGE SAUCE

Servings
2

Protein per serving..........8 oz/225 g
Carbohydrate per serving...........11 g

¼ cup onion, finely diced

2 oz /60 g butter

1 tsp all purpose/plain flour

¼ cup beef or chicken stock

¼ cup dry white wine

¼ cup orange juice

⇨Melt half butter in a small saucepan and sauté onions until tender. Do not brown.

⇨Sprinkle with flour and stir for 2 minutes.

⇨Stir in stock, wine and orange juice. Bring to boil, reduce heat, cover and simmer for 20 minutes.

4 pork loin chops each 4 oz/110 g

Salt and pepper to taste

1 tsp French mustard

1 tsp parsley, chopped

⇨Melt remaining butter in skillet or pan. Season both sides of chops with salt and pepper. Sear chops in hot pan, reduce heat and sauté until just cooked.

⇨Arrange chops on plates. Beat mustard into sauce and spoon over chops. Garnish with parsley.

BAVARIAN PORK CHOPS

Servings
2

Protein per serving..........8 oz/225 g
Carbohydrate per serving..............5 g

4 pork loin chops each 4 oz/110 g

Salt and pepper to taste

1 TBL all purpose/plain flour

½ cup dry white wine

1 cup mushrooms, sliced

¼ cup sour cream

⇨Trim fat from chops, heat in hot skillet or pan until it melts. Discard solids.

⇨Put flour, salt and pepper in paper or plastic bag and dredge chops.

⇨Sear chops on both sides in hot pan. Pour off excess fat and add wine. Cover and simmer until cooked.

⇨Remove from pan and add mushrooms. Simmer 5 minutes.

⇨Remove mushrooms from pan, reduce liquid by half and add sour cream and spoon sauce over chops.

OSSOBUCCO

Servings
3

Protein per serving..........8 oz/225 g
Carbohydrate per serving..............6 g

2 lb/900 g shin veal, cut through bone in 1 in/25 mm slices

2 TBL all purpose/plain flour

Salt and pepper to taste

2 TBL olive oil

1 bay leaf

1 garlic clove, crushed

1 cup onion, sliced

1 cup celery, sliced

1 TBL butter

1 cup tomatoes, canned

¼ tsp basil, dried

¼ cup red wine

3 cups beef stock

1 parsley sprig, chopped

⇨Mix flour, salt and pepper in paper or plastic bag. Dredge veal pieces.

⇨Heat oil in skillet or pan, add sage and garlic and lightly brown veal pieces.

⇨Remove veal to ovenproof dish. Add butter, onion and celery to pan and sauté till tender.

⇨Add tomato, basil, wine and bay leaf and simmer for 10 minutes.

⇨Pour sauce over meat and add stock. Cook in moderate oven for 90 minutes.

⇨Arrange meat on serving dish, top with sauce and garnish with chopped parsley.

LAMB

LAMB CUTLETS WITH PIQUANT SAUCE

Servings
2

Protein per serving..........8 oz/225 g
Carbohydrate per serving..............8 g

6 lamb cutlets each 3 oz/85 g

¼ cup all purpose/plain flour

1 egg

¼ cup milk

¼cup toasted bread crumbs

¼ cup olive oil

Sauce

1 TBL onion, finely chopped

1 tsp parsley, chopped

1 tsp capers, finely chopped

1 anchovy fillet, mashed

¼ cup mayonnaise

Dash Worcestershire sauce

⅛ teaspoon mustard

⮞Combine sauce ingredients in a mixing bowl and chill.

⮞Lightly beat egg and milk together in a bowl.

⮞Dredge cutlets in flour, dip in egg mixture and lightly cover with bread crumbs.

⮞Heat oil in skillet or pan and sauté cutlets on both sides over low heat until golden brown.

⮞Serve with piquant sauce.

BARBECUED LAMB WITH HONEY AND LEMON

Servings
2

Protein per serving..........8 oz/225 g
Carbohydrate per serving..............5 g

4 lamb leg chops each 4 oz/110 g

Salt and pepper to taste

Marinade

2 TBL olive oil

3 TBL lemon juice

1 TBL honey

1 garlic clove, crushed

2 bay leaves, crushed

⇨Season chops with salt and pepper and place in shallow dish.

⇨Combine marinade ingredients in a separate bowl and pour over chops.

⇨Cover and refrigerate for 4 hours, turning chops occasionally.

⇨Broil, grill or barbecue chops while occasionally basting with marinade.

RACK OF LAMB WITH CRANBERRY SAUCE

Servings
2

Protein per serving..........8 oz/225 g
Carbohydrate per serving..............8 g

2 racks of lamb each with four chops

Salt and pepper to taste

2 TBL cranberries, canned

1 tsp rosemary, dried

⇨Remove excess fat from lamb and score skin with sharp knife to overcome shrinkage.

⇨Season lamb with salt and pepper and spread cranberry on meat with a knife. Sprinkle with rosemary.

⇨Bake in moderate oven for 40 minutes or until lamb is cooked.

⇨Slice into cutlets and serve.

IRISH STEW

Servings
3

Protein per serving..........8 oz/225 g
Carbohydrate per serving...........18 g

2 lb/900 g lamb neck or shoulder chops	⇨Put flour, salt and pepper in plastic or paper bag and dredge chops.
2 TBL all purpose/plain flour	
Salt and pepper to taste	⇨Heat oil in large saucepan, sauté onions and garlic but do not brown. Remove from pan.
2 TBL olive oil	
1 cup onion, sliced	⇨Brown chops on both sides and add onion, carrot, potato, herbs and stock or water.
1 garlic clove, crushed	
1 cup carrot, sliced	
8 oz/220 g potato, peeled and quartered	⇨Cover and simmer for 80 minutes. Remove lid and reduce liquid to form a thin sauce.
½ tsp oregano, dried	
½ tsp basil, dried	⇨Serve.
2 cups stock or water	

BEEF

BRAISED STEAK AND KIDNEY

Servings
4

Protein per serving..........8 oz/225 g
Carbohydrate per serving..............6 g

1¼ lb/800 g topside or round steak, cubed	⇨Remove skin and fat from kidneys. Cube and soak in cold salty water for 30 minutes. Drain.
4 lamb or 1 beef or veal kidney	
2 TBL all purpose/plain flour	⇨Season flour with salt and pepper. Dredge beef and kidney in flour mixture.
Salt and pepper to taste	
2 TBL olive oil	⇨Heat oil in heavy saucepan sauté onion and garlic until tender. Do not brown.
1 onion, sliced	
2 garlic cloves, crushed	⇨Remove onion from oil and brown beef and kidney. Add residual flour and stir for 3 minutes.
2 cups stock or water	
1 TBL tomato ketchup	⇨Stir in cold stock or water and add sauces and herbs.
Dash Worcestershire sauce	
¼ tsp oregano, dried	⇨Simmer covered for 2 hours and serve.
¼ tsp basil, dried	

MEAT BALLS PARMESAN

Servings
2

Protein per serving..........8 oz/225 g
Carbohydrate per serving...........16 g

1 lb/440 g ground/minced beef	⇨Combine beef, garlic, bread crumbs, cheese and parsley and form into balls
2 garlic cloves, crushed	
1 slice bread, crumbled	⇨Toss meat balls in flour seasoned with salt and pepper.
¼ cup parmesan cheese, grated	

2 parsley sprigs, chopped

2 TBL all purpose/plain flour

Salt and pepper to taste

¼ cup olive oil

1 cup prepared Italian tomato sauce

¼ cup red or white wine

⇨Heat oil in skillet or pan and fry meat balls until brown. Do not cook through.

⇨Arrange meat balls in a covered ovenproof dish and add wine and Italian sauce.

⇨Bake in moderate oven for 30 minutes and serve.

ORIENTAL SLICED BEEF

Servings
2

Protein per serving..........8 oz/225 g
Carbohydrate per serving..........1.5 g

2 steaks each 8 oz/220 g

3 TBL soy sauce

1 TBL oyster sauce

1 TBL fish sauce (nam pla)

1 garlic clove, crushed

½ cup water

⇨Combine sauces and garlic in bowl and marinate meat for 2 hours.

⇨Barbecue or broil to desired doneness and slice.

⇨Add water to remaining marinade and simmer in saucepan while steaks are cooking.

⇨Serve with steamed broccoli and rice (not included in nutrient assessment) and use sauce as a dip.

STEAK DIANE

Servings
2

Protein per serving..........8 oz/225 g
Carbohydrate per serving..............3 g

2 fillet or rib eye steaks each 8 oz/220 g	⇨Season steaks with salt and pepper.
Salt and pepper to taste	⇨Melt butter in skillet or pan, add garlic and fry steaks until brown on both sides.
1 oz/30 g butter	
1 garlic clove, crushed	
¼ tsp lemon zest	⇨Add lemon zest, chives, Worcestershire sauce and brandy. When hot, ignite brandy.
1 TBL chives, chopped	
3 tsp Worcestershire sauce	⇨When cooked, remove steaks and add cream to pan. Cook sauce for 1 minute and spoon over steaks.
2 TBL brandy	
¼ cup cream	

carbohydrate assessment chart

The following chart contains the approximate carbohydrate content of most common foods and beverages. The carbohydrate content of any food or food product may vary between manufacturers, geographical areas of planting, or seasons. However, the total carbohydrate content of a cross-section of foods and beverages will usually average out to be sufficiently accurate for the purpose of assessing your daily carbohydrate intake.

Except where otherwise specified, the carbohydrate content of each product is stated as grams for both the metric and the imperial measuring systems. The use of ounces of carbohydrate in most cases would be inappropriate because of the relative size of an ounce when compared to a gram. As one ounce is equal to 28 grams, the carbohydrate content of many products would have to be stated in fractions of an ounce. This would make the assessment of the majority of foods and beverages extremely difficult.

Irrespective of the measuring system you choose you can remove any confusion by thinking of grams of carbohydrate simply as being *units* of carbohydrate.

When assessing the carbohydrate content of any product, it is not the weight of the product that is important. The carbohydrate count is the amount of carbohydrate or sugar contained in a specific quantity of a particular product. In most cases the carbohydrate content of a product is stated in grams (or units) per 100 g of product, and again in grams (or units) per ounce of product.

The carbohdrate content of each product is given to the nearest 0.5 g, but you may choose multiples or fractions of the amounts given. For example, as asparagus is given in multiples of 100 g, your choice of 200 g of asparagus would simply mean doubling the given amount in the metric column. Or, if you choose less than 100 g of a particular product, for instance, 25 g of curry powder, you would divide the amount given in the metric column by four. A similar amount of asparagus in the imperial measuring system would be 7 oz, therefore, you would multiply the amount given in the imperial column by seven. Twenty five grams of curry powder is approximately equal to 1 oz, therefore you would simply calculate the amount as stated in the imperial column.

For ease of assessment all foods and beverages have been listed under their relative group headings. Both the group heading and the individual foods and beverages contained in each group are listed in alphabetical order.

CARBOHYDRATE ASSESSMENT CHART

TABLE OF CONTENTS

CARBOHYDRTE ASSESSMENT CHART

BEVERAGES	Measure	Carbohydrate (g)
Alcoholic		
beer, ale	10 fl oz/300 ml	12
lager	10 fl oz/300 ml	12
light	10 fl oz/300 ml	7.5
brandy	1.5 fl oz/45 ml	2.5
bourbon	1.5 fl oz/45 ml	1.5
cider, dry	10 fl oz/300 ml	18
sweet	10 fl oz/300 ml	23
gin	1.5 fl oz/45 ml	2
port	1.5 fl oz/45 ml	8
rum	1.5 fl oz/45 ml	1.5
sherry	1.5 fl oz/45 ml	6
stout	10 fl oz/300 ml	12
vermouth, dry	1.5 fl oz/45 ml	6
sweet	1.5 fl oz/45 ml	8
vodka	1.5 fl oz/45 ml	1.5
whisky	1.5 fl oz/45 ml	2
wine, table	3.5 fl oz/100 ml	6
Non-alcoholic		
chicory	8 fl oz/240 ml	63
cocoa, made with milk	8 fl oz/240 ml	27
cola, regular	10 fl oz/300 ml	33
diet	10 fl oz/300 ml	0.5
coffee, black, unsweetened	8 fl oz/240 ml	trace
creamed, unsweetened	8 fl oz/240 ml	1.5
dry ginger ale	0 fl oz/300 ml	11.5
ginger beer	10 fl oz/300 ml	31
malted milk	8 fl oz/240 ml	27
milk, whole	8 fl oz/240 ml	12
mineral water	10 fl oz/300 ml	0
soda water	10 fl oz/300 ml	0
soft drinks (average)	10 fl oz/300 ml	30
root beer	10 fl oz/300 ml	32
tea - black, unsweetened	8 fl oz/240 ml	trace
with milk, unsweetened	8 fl oz/240 ml	0.5
Tom Collins mix	8 fl oz/240 ml	30
tonic water	10 fl oz/300 ml	20

	Per 100 g	Per oz
BREAD		
brown	46	13
cracked wheat	52	15
crumbs	73	21
currant	52	15
French	55	16
Hovis	68	19
Italian	56	16
malt	49	14
pumpernickel	53	15
raisin	53	15
rolls, enriched	57	16.5
rye	52	15
Vienna	55	16
white, enriched	50	14
whole wheat	49	14
BREAKFAST CEREALS		
All Bran	43	12
Cornflakes	85	24
farina, cooked	9	2.5
grapenuts	76	22
muesli	66	19
oatmeal/rolled oats	9.5	3
puffed wheat	80	23
Quakers oats, raw	67	19
Rice Krispies	88	25
shredded wheat	80	23
Special K	78	22
Weetbix	70	20
wheat flakes	80	23
wheat germ	53	15
CAKES, COOKIES AND CRACKERS		
Cakes		
angelfood	59	17
Boston cream pie	49	14
coconut	53	15
muffins, corn	50	14
white flour	42	12
cupcakes, iced	56	16
chocolate icing	77	22

	Per 100 g	Per oz
currant	64	18
Danish pastry	46	13
devil's food, iced	58	17
doughnuts, plain	50	14
fruitcake	60	17
gingerbread	51	15
pancakes, plain	33	9.5
buckwheat	22	6.5
plain, without icing	56	16
iced	62	18
pound	47	13.5
sponge, plain	54	15.5
with jam	64	18
Welsh cheesecake	60	17
white layer, iced	63	18
yellow, without icing	58	17
iced	60	17

Cookies

brownies, with nuts	65	18.5
chocolate	67	19
chocolate chip	50	14
cream slices	70	20
fig bars	79	22.5
ginger snaps	79	22.5
plain	70	20
shortbread	65	18
vanilla wafers	66	19

Crackers

cheddar	55	16
crispbread, starch reduced	37	10
rye	71	20
Graham	71	20
Ryvita	66	19
Saltines	69	20
Vita-Weat	78	22
water	76	21

DAIRY PRODUCTS

butter	trace	trace
buttermilk, cultured	5	1.5
dried	50	14
cheese, American processed	7	2
blue and roquefort	trace	trace

	Per 100 g	Per oz
Camembert	trace	trace
cheddar	trace	trace
cottage	3	1
cream	2	0.5
parmesan	3.5	1
Swiss	3.5	1
spread, American	7	2
spread, English	1	trace
cream, fresh	3	1
imitation, liquid	10	3
imitatiom, powdered	55	16
sour, fresh	4.5	1
immitation	1.5	0.5
whipped topping, canned	10	3
ice-cream, regular (10% fat)	21	6
rich (16% fat)	18	5
iced milk, hardened	22.5	6.5
soft-serve	22	6.5
milk, full cream	5	1.5
buttermilk	4	1
condensed, sweetened	54	15.5
evaporated, unsweetened	10	3
nonfat, skimmed	5	1.5
2% fat	6	1.5
powder, full cream	39	11
low fat	53	15
yoghurt, natural	5.5	1.5
flavoured	14	4
fruit	18	5
hazelnut	16	5
natural	5.5	1.5

DESSERTS

apple crumble	37	10
apple dumpling	29	8
apple pudding	30	8
apple stewed, sweetened	17	5
unsweetened	8	3
custard, baked	15	4
banana	18	5
pie, apple	38	11
butterscotch	38	11
cherry	38	11

	Per 100 g	Per oz
custard	23	6.5
fruit mince	42	12
lemon meringue	38	11
pecan	51	14.5
pineapple chiffon	39	11
pumpkin	25	7
piecrust	44	12.5
pudding, chocolate	26	7.5
vanilla (blanc mange)	16	4.5
sherbet	30	9
tapioca, with apple	30	9
cream pudding	17	5

EGGS

	Per 100 g	Per oz
egg, large 2 oz/60 gm	trace	trace
white	trace	trace
yolk	trace	trace
scrambled with milk	1	trace

FAST FOOD

Kentucky Fried Chicken

	Per 100 g	Per oz
bean salad	21	6
burger, (stated in grams of carbohydrate per item)		
chicken fillet	31	
with bacon & cheese	35	
the works	42	
coleslaw	13.5	4
gravy	4.5	1
KFC original recipe (bone included)*	6	1.5
nuggets	11	3
potato, mashed with gravy	12.5	3.5
potato salad	18 5	

*(average bone content of Kentucky Fried Chicken is 25% of total cooked weight)

McDonald's

(stated in grams of carbohydrate per item to nearest half gram)

Junior burger	29
Cheeseburger	26
Quarter pounder with cheese	33
McFeast	29.5
Big Mac	40

McChicken	39
Filet-O-Fish	44
Chicken McNuggets, each	2
Big Breakfast	48
hotcakes, butter and syrup	91
bacon and egg McMuffin	24
sausage McMuffin	25
sausage McMuffin with egg	27
scrambled eggs & muffin	24
English muffin, butter & jam	37
hash brown's	16
fries, small	19
medium	30
large	37.5
apple and oatbran muffin	45
apple pie	26
McDonaldland cookies	40.5
sundae, hot fudge	41
strawberry	43
caramel	37.5
barbeque sauce	12.5
mild curry sauce	11
sweet mustard sauce	6.5
sweet and sour sauce	13.5
milk shake, chocolate	44.5
strawberry	48.5
vanilla	38.5

Pizza Hut (the carbohdrate content of each item is per medium slice)

Pan Pizza

Super Supreme	35.5
Supreme	32
Hawaiian	36
Cheese	29

Thin 'N Crispy Pizza

Super Supreme	26
Supreme	27
Hawaiian	26.5
Cheese	21.5

FATS AND OILS

	Per 100 g	Per oz
lard	0	0
margarine	trace	trace
oleo (beef)	0	0
vegetable	0	0

FLOUR AND GRAIN PRODUCTS

Flour

all purpose/plain	71	20
buckwheat	80	23
self-raising	75	21
whole-wheat	71	20
corn starch/flour	92	25

Grain products

chapatis	44	12
cornmeal, bolted or unbolted	74	21
degermed	78	22.5
crumpets	37	10
hominy (grits)	11	3
macaroni, boiled	28	8
pie crust, white flour	50	14
pasta, boiled	23	6.5
popcorn, plain	63	18
rice, polished, raw	81	23
polished, boiled	24	7
instant	24	7
semolina, raw	78	22
creamed	11	3
pudding	20	6
waffles	37	11

FRUIT

apple, cooking	10	3
eating	12	3.5
applesauce, unsweetened	11	3
sweetened	24	7
apricots, fresh	12	3.5
in heavy syrup	22	6
dried	67	19
avocado	8	2

	Per 100 g	Per oz
bananas, fresh	15	4
dried	89	25.5
blackberries	15	4
blackcurrants	6	2
blueberries	15	4
cantaloupe	3.5	1
cherries	12	4
chestnuts, shelled	37	10
cranberries	4	1
currants, dried	63	18
dates, pitted	73	21
figs, fresh	10	3
dried	71	20
gooseberries	3	1
grapefruit, fresh	5	1.5
canned in syrup	18	5
frozen concentrate	35	10
grapes, slip skin	10	3
tight skin	16	4.5
lemons	6	1.5
limes	9	2.5
loganberries	3	1
lychees	16	5
mango	12	4
orange	9	2.5
papaya	10	3
passion fruit	3	1
peaches, fresh	9	2.5
in heavy syrup	20	6
dried	68	19.5
pears, fresh	14	4
in heavy syrup	20	6
pineapple, fresh	14	4
in heavy syrup	19	5.5
plums, fresh	12	4
in heavy syrup	21	6
prunes, dried	56	16
cooked, unsweetened	29	8
quince, fresh	6	2
raisins, seedless	79	22
raspberries, fresh	14	4
frozen	25	7
rhubarb, stewed, unsweetened	1	trace
stewed, sweetened	11	1
rockmelon	3.5	1

	Per 100 g	Per oz
strawberries, fresh	9	2.5
frozen	28	8
tangerine	9	3
watermelon, including rind	3	1

JUICES, FRUIT AND VEGETABLE

	Per 100 g	Per oz
apple	12	3.5
apricot nectar	15	4
cranberry coctail	17	5
grapefruit, unsweetened	9	2.7
sweetened	13	3.5
concentrate	35	10
grape, fresh	17	5
concentrate	46	13
juice drink	14	4
lemonade, concentrate	51	14.5
limeade, concentrate	50	14
orange, fresh	10.5	3
concentrate	41	11.5
orange-apricot juice drink	13	3.5
orange & grapefruit, concentrate	37	10.5
pineapple	14	4
prune	19	5.5
tangerine, canned sweetened	12	3.5
tomato	4	1

MEAT (BEEF, GAME, LAMB, PORK, POULTRY AND VEAL)

Fresh Meats

	Per 100 g	Per oz
bacon	0	0
beef, all cuts	0	0
ground	0	0
hamburger, meat only	0	0
brains	0	0
chicken	0	0
duck	0	0
game	0	0
goose	0	0
heart, beef	1	trace
kidneys, all types	0	0
lamb, all cuts	0	0
liver, all types	4	1
pork, all cuts	0	0
sweetbreads, fried	6	2
veal, all cuts	0	0

	Per 100 g	Per oz
Prepared Meats		
bologna	trace	trace
bratwurst	0	0
brawn	0	0
corned beef, fresh	0	0
canned	0	0
hash	11	3
frankfurter	3	1
ham, on bone	0	0
deviled	0	0
salami	trace	trace
sausage, beef with filler	15	4.5
black	15	4.5
liver	4	1
luncheon	5	1.5
pork, with filler	11	3
pork links	trace	trace
Vienna	trace	trace
saveloy	10	3
MISCELLANEOUS ITEMS		
baking powder	38	11
barbecue sauce	8	2
bouillon cubes	trace	trace
chicory, raw	2	1
chutney, apple	50	14
sweet mango	60	17
tomato	40	11.5
cranberry sauce, sweetened	37	11
gelatin	0	0
honey	76	22
mayonnaise	0	0
meat extract	3	1
nutmeat, granose	11	3
brawn	5	1.5
pretzels	75	21
salt	0	0
tartare sauce	7	2
tomato, catsup	25	7
puree	11	3
sauce	8	3
treacle	67	19
vinegar	7	2

	Per 100 g	Per oz

NUTS AND DRY LEGUMES

	Per 100 g	Per oz
almonds, shelled	20	6
beans, great northern	21	6
navy	21	6
red kidney, canned	16.5	5
lima	26	7.5
cashews	29	8.5
coconut, dried	9	2.5
cowpeas/blackeye peas	13.5	4
peanuts, roasted	19	5.5
butter, pure	19	5.5
peas, dried split	21	6
pecans	15	4
walnuts	15	4

PREPARED MEALS

	Per 100 g	Per oz
beef pot pie	19	5.5
beefsteak pie	21	6
beefsteak pudding	19	5
beef stew	4	1
beef & vegetable stew	6.5	2
chicken casserole	21	6
chicken curry	8	3
chicken pot pie	18.5	5
chilli con carne, with beans	12	3.5
without beans	6	1.5
Cornish pasties	31	9
cottage pie	9	3
Irish stew	7	2
Lancashire hot-pot	10	3
meatballs in gravy	6	2
moussaka	10	3
pork pie	25	7
Scotch egg	12	3

SEAFOOD

	Per 100 g	Per oz
calamari	0	0
clams, fresh	2	0.5
canned including liquid	2	0.5
crabmeat, fresh	0	0
canned	1	trace
fish, breaded	7	2

	Per 100 g	Per oz
fish, white	0	0
fish sticks/fingers, breaded	14	4
mussels	trace	trace
oysters, raw	trace	trace
prawns, fresh	0	0
roe, fried	3	1
salmon, fresh	0	0
scallops	trace	trace
scampi, broiled	0	0
battered	29	8
shrimp, canned	1	trace
tuna, fresh or canned	0	0

SOUPS

cream of chicken	6	1.5
cream of mushroom	6	1.5
cream of oyster	6	1.5
cream of potato	7	2
cream of shrimp	6	1.5
cream of tomato	9	2.5
bean with pork	9	2.5
beef broth	1	trace
beef noodle	3	1
clam chowder	5	1.5
minestrone	6	1.5
split pea	9	2.5
vegetable beef	4	1
vegetarian	5	1.5

SUGAR, CANDY, JAMS AND SYRUPS

cake icing, chocolate	67	19
coconut	75	21.5
fudge	75	21.5
white, boiled	81	23
caramels	79	22.5
chocolate, milk, plain	56	16
fancy	73	21
fruit and nut	51	15
with nuts	48	14
fondant	88	25
fudge	74	21
golden syrup	79	22
gum drops	88	25

	Per 100 g	Per oz
hard candy	98	28
honey	55	16
jams and preserves	70	20
jello/jellies	72	20.5
marshmallows	81	23
molasses	65	18.5
sugar, brown	96	27.5
powdered	100	28.5
white	100	28.5
syrup, corn	72	20.5
sorgum	67	19
topping	84	24

VEGETABLES

	Per 100 g	Per oz
asparagus, fresh, boiled	1	0.5
canned	3	1
artichoke, boiled	3	1
aubergine	3	1
beans, broad, raw	14	4
boiled	7	2
butter, raw	50	14
boiled	17	5
French, boiled	1	0.5
green runner, boiled	3	1
green snap, boiled	6	1.5
haricot, boiled	17	5
lima, boiled	0.5	trace
red kidney	45	13
sprouts, mung	6	1.5
yellow or wax, boiled	5	1.5
beets/beetroot, boiled	7	2
canned	8	2
greens, boiled	3.5	1
blackeye peas/cowpeas	0.5	trace
broccoli, boiled	2	0.5
brussels sprouts, boiled	2	1
cabbage, raw	4	1
boiled	1	0.5
capsicum	5.5	1.5
carrots, raw	5	1.5
boiled	4	1
cauliflower, raw	2	1
boiled	1	0.5

	Per 100 g	Per oz
celery, raw	2	1
boiled	1	0.5
chives	0	0
collards	5	1.5
corn, boiled, on cob	11	3
canned	16	4.5
cress	trace	trace
cucumber, raw	3.5	1
pickled, dill	1.5	0.5
sweet, gherkin	40	11
sweet, relish	33	9.5
dandelion greens, boiled	7	2
eggplant	3	1
endive	3.5	1
kale, boiled	4	1
leeks, raw	6	2
boiled	5	1
lettuce	2	0.5
mint, fresh	39	11
mushrooms, fresh	0	0
canned	2.5	1
mustard greens, boiled	4	1
okra, boiled	6	1.5
olives, pickled	trace	trace
onion	7	2
onion, green/shallot	10	3
parsley	trace	trace
parsnips, boiled	14	4
peas, green, fresh	11	3
boiled	8	2
frozen, boiled	4	1
canned	12	3.5
peppers, hot, red	53	15
peppers, sweet, bell	5.5	1.5
potato, baked	25	7
boiled, new	18	5
boiled, old	20	6
chipped (English)	37	11
chips (American)	49	14
crisps (English)	49	14
French fries (American)	37	11
instant	16	5
mashed	18	5
sweet, boiled	33	9.5

	Per 100 g	Per oz
candied	34	10
roast, old	27	8
tinned, new	13	4
pumpkin, fresh	3	1
canned	9	2
radish	3	1
sauerkraut, canned	4	1
spinach	3	1
spring greens	1	trace
squash, summer, boiled	3	1
winter, baked	16	4.5
swedes, boiled	4	1
tomatoes, raw	3	1
canned	4	1
turnips, boiled	5	1.5
greens, boiled	3.5	1
watercress	1	trace
yams, boiled	30	9

bibliography

Ardrey, R., *African Genesis – A Personal Investigation into the Animal Origins and Nature of Man*, Dell Publishing Co. Inc., New York, 1967: 181.

Department of Community Services and Health, *National Dietary Survey of School Children (10–15 years)*, 1985.

Erdmann, R. and Jones, M., *Fats Nutrition and Health*, Thorsons Publishing Group, Northamptonshire, England, 1990.

Everson, J., 'What's the best fuel for muscles', *Muscle & Fitness*, Weider Publishing, Gymea, June 1990.

Frazer, J., 'Exercise your right to never say diet', *The Weekend Australian – Review*, March 21-22, 1992: 1.

Giedion S., *Mechanization Takes Command*, Oxford University Press, New York, 1948.

Giller, R. M. and Mathews, K., *Medical Makeover*, Beech Tree Books, William Morrow and Company Inc., New York, 1986.

Gittleman, A. L., *Beyond Pritikin*, Bantam Books, New York, 1989.

Gitterson, B., *Biorhythm – A Personal Science*, Futura Publications Limited, London, 1976.

Goodhart, R.S. and Shils, M. E., *Modern Nutrition in Health and Disease – Dietotherapy*, 5th ed, Lea & Febiger, Philadelphia, 1976.

Grant, D., *Your Daily Food*, Faber and Faber, London, 1973.

Guthrie, H. A., *Introductory Nutrition*, The C.V. Mosby Company, Saint Louis, 1975: 197.

Guyton, A.C., *Textbook Of Medical Physiology*, W.B. Saunders Company, Philadelphia, 1976.

Hall, R. H., *Food for Nought – The Decline in Nutrition*, Harper & Row, New York, 1974.

Haymaker, W. and Anderson, E., 'Disorders of the hypothalamus and pituitary gland', *Clinical Neurology* Vol 2, Ch 28, Harper & Row, Hagerstown, 1975.

Luoma, T.C., 'Quick Facts', *Ironman*, Fitness Publications Ltd., Aston, March 1993.

Mayer, J., 'Obesity', *Modern Nutrition in Health and Disease – Dietotherapy*, 5th ed, Ch 22, Lea & Febiger, Philadelphia, 1976: 642.

Orten, J.M. and Neuhaus, O.W., *Human Biochemistry*, 9th ed, The C.V. Mosby Company, Saint Louis, 1975.

Robbins, S.L., *Pathologic Basis Of Disease*, W.B. Saunders Company, Philadelphia, 1974.

Stewart, M., *Beat Sugar Craving*, Vermilion, London, 1992.

United States Department of Agriculture, 'Nutritive values of the edible parts of foods', *Home and Garden Bulletin* No. 72, Washington D.C., 1970.

United States Department of Health, Education and Welfare, 'Healthy People: The Surgeon General's report on health promotion and disease prevention', 1979.

United States Senate Committee on Commerce, Consumer Subcommittee, *Dry Cereal Hearings*, Ninety-first Congress, Second Session, serial No 91-72, 23 July, 4, 5 August 1970.

United States Senate Select Committee on Foodstuffs, *Eggs and the AHA*, 10 September 1973.

United States Senate Select Committee on Nutrition and Human Needs, Part 3, 12 March 1973.

Williams, S.R., *Nutrition and diet therapy*, The C.V. Mosby Company, Saint Louis 1977: 477.